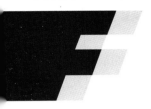

FAST FACTS

Indispensable

Guides to

Clinical

Practice

Diabetes Mellitus

Ian W Campbell

Honorary Professor, Department of Biological
and Medical Sciences, University of St
Andrews, and Consultant Physician, Victoria
Hospital, Kirkcaldy, Fife, UK

Harold Lebovitz

Professor of Medicine, Chief Section of
Endocrinology, State University of New York
Health Science Center at Brooklyn, New York,
USA

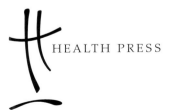

HEALTH PRESS

Oxford

Fast Facts – Diabetes Mellitus
First Published 1996

© 1996 Health Press
Elizabeth House, Queen Street, Abingdon,
Oxford, UK OX14 3JR
Tel: +44 (0)1235 523233
Fax: +44 (0)1235 523238

Professor IW Campbell wishes to acknowledge
Dr AC MacCuish, Dr CJ Bailey, Dr JM Steel,
Dr PJ Leslie and Dr M Macdonald for their
support.

A CIP catalogue record for this title is available
from the British Library.

ISBN 1-899541-35-7

Library of Congress
Cataloguing-in-Publication Data

Campbell, I. (Ian)
Fast Facts – Diabetes Mellitus/
Ian Campbell, Harold Lebovitz

Designed and typeset by Hinton Chaundy
Design Partnership, Thame, UK

Printed by Spectrum Press (Northampton)
Limited, Northampton, UK

Glossary

CAPD: chronic ambulatory peritoneal dialysis

Euglycaemic clamp: a technique for measuring insulin sensitivity

Glycosylated haemoglobin: glycated haemoglobin (see below)

Glycated haemoglobin (HbA_1/HbA_{1C}): an indicator of glycaemic control, that reflects control during the previous 4–6 weeks

Gustatory sweating: sweating provoked by food (a manifestation of autonomic neuropathy)

HLA: histocompatibility antigens

ICA: islet cell antibodies

IDDM: insulin-dependent diabetes mellitus

Indirect fluorescence: a technique for detection of islet cell antibodies

Insulin resistance syndrome: an alternative name for metabolic syndrome

Metabolic syndrome: a syndrome consisting of insulin resistance, hyperinsulinaemia, glucose intolerance, hypertension, dyslipidaemia and obesity, commonly found in patients with NIDDM

NIDDM: non-insulin dependent diabetes mellitus

Radioimmunoassay: an analytical technique that can be used to measure circulating concentrations of insulin, proinsulin and C–peptide

Reaven's syndrome: an alternative name for metabolic syndrome

Somogyi effect: the combination of nocturnal hypoglycaemia and fasting hyperglycaemia

Syndrome X: an alternative name for metabolic syndrome

CHAPTER 1

Epidemiology

Diabetes mellitus is now recognized as a major worldwide public health problem. At present, about 100 million people have diabetes mellitus and the prevalence is rising, especially in developing countries as they become more Westernized. Indeed, by the year 2010, it has been estimated that there will be over 200 million people with diabetes mellitus throughout the world.

Three main types of diabetes mellitus are recognized.

- Insulin-dependent diabetes mellitus (IDDM) or type I diabetes mellitus accounts for 5–25% of cases, depending on ethnic background.
- Non-insulin-dependent diabetes mellitus (NIDDM) or type 2 diabetes mellitus accounts for 75–90% of cases depending on ethnic background.
- Diabetes mellitus secondary to certain medical conditions or associated with genetic syndromes (Table 1.1) accounts for approximately 1–5% of cases.

TABLE 1.1

Causes of secondary diabetes mellitus

Endocrine

- Acromegaly
- Cushing's syndrome
- Phaeochromocytoma
- Hyperthyroidism

Pancreatic

- Pancreatectomy
- Chronic pancreatitis
- Carcinoma
- Haemochromatosis

Drug-induced

- Corticosteroids
- Thiazides
- β-blockers

Genetic syndromes

- Down's syndrome
- DIDMOAD (diabetes insipidus, diabetes mellitus, optic atrophy, deafness)

Hepatic

- Cirrhosis

Prevalence

The prevalence of diabetes mellitus in Western countries has traditionally been estimated to be 2–6%, of which half of the patients are diagnosed and a similar number unrecognized. However, this figure is now known to be much higher in older people and non-whites. Probably 10–20% of individuals over the age of 65 are affected. In the non-white populations living in a Western culture (e.g. Asians in the UK, Pacific Islanders, Pima Indians) as many as 15–20% of the total population have diabetes (Table 1.2).

TABLE 1.2

Effects of race and age on prevalence of diabetes mellitus in Western cultures[1]

	Age	
	20–44 years	45–74 years
Non-Hispanic white	1.6%	12.0%
Black	3.3%	19.3%
Mexican Americans	3.8%	23.9%
Pima Indians	40%	65%
South-Asian Indians	16–20%	

[1]Data from Harris M, ed. *Diabetes in America*. 2nd ed. New York: US Department of Health and Human Services, 1995.

Mortality and morbidity

Before the introduction of insulin 75 years ago, young IDDM patients died within 1–3 years from diabetic coma (diabetic ketoacidosis) and, indeed, this may still happen in developing countries with a shortage of drugs. In general, however, this appalling prognosis has dramatically changed with the advent of insulin therapy and oral anti-hyperglycaemic drugs. Although life expectancy has subsequently increased, this has been accompanied by a considerable rise in the incidence of chronic complications, both microvascular (retinopathy, nephropathy and neuropathy) and macrovascular (cardiac, cerebral and peripheral vascular), which have now become the principal cause of morbidity and mortality in diabetes mellitus.

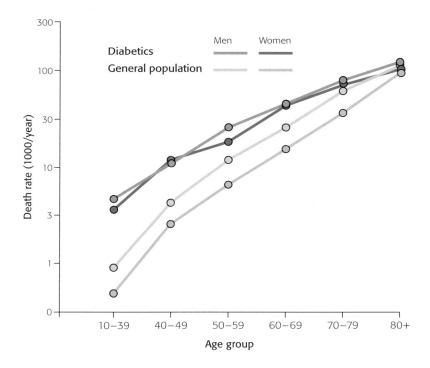

Figure 1.1 The results of a prospective mortality study carried out in Edinburgh, UK, demonstrate the increased mortality rate in both men and women with diabetes mellitus compared with the general population. (Data from Shenfield GM et al. *Diabete Metab (Paris)* 1979; 5:149–158.)

The mortality rate in patients with diabetes mellitus is higher than that in the general population (Figure 1.1) and life expectancy in both IDDM and NIDDM is reduced by about 8–10 years. In contrast to the general population, the mortality rate among female diabetic patients is virtually identical to that in males, and the increased mortality is mainly attributable to cardiovascular disease and renal failure.

The morbidity and premature mortality seen in both IDDM and NIDDM is putting increasing pressure on healthcare resources. Early diagnosis of diabetes mellitus is important, especially in NIDDM, where the diagnosis may be delayed and complications unfortunately present at the time of diagnosis. The Diabetes Control and Complications Trial (DCCT) in the

TABLE 1.3

The St Vincent Declaration (1989) – 5-year targets for Europe

- To reduce new blindness due to diabetes mellitus by 30% or more
- To reduce the number of patients entering end-stage diabetic renal failure by at least 30%
- To reduce the rate of limb amputations for diabetic gangrene by 50%
- To cut morbidity and mortality from coronary heart disease and stroke by vigorous programmes of risk factor reduction
- To achieve a pregnancy outcome in diabetic women that approximates to that in non-diabetic women

USA has shown that in IDDM, good glycaemic control can prevent microvascular and neuropathic complications or delay their progression. The early detection of retinopathy, nephropathy and neuropathy can lead to a reduction in the incidence of blindness, kidney failure and amputation due to diabetes mellitus. In recognition of this, the St Vincent Declaration has set 5-year targets in Europe, which are currently being implemented, to reduce both the microvascular and macrovascular complications of diabetes mellitus (Table 1.3).

CHAPTER 2

What is IDDM?

IDDM results from the progressive destruction of β-cells in the islets of Langerhans, which leads to insulin deficiency (Figure 2.1). The symptoms of diabetes mellitus become apparent when approximately 80–85% of the β-cells have been lost. Thus, although the symptoms of IDDM usually have a relatively sudden onset, the underlying pathophysiological changes occur over a prolonged period. β-cell destruction appears to be an autoimmune reaction, which can be triggered by a variety of environmental factors, and individuals who develop IDDM are those with a genetic susceptibility to activate this autoimmune process (Figure 2.2). The characteristic features of IDDM are summarized in Table 2.1.

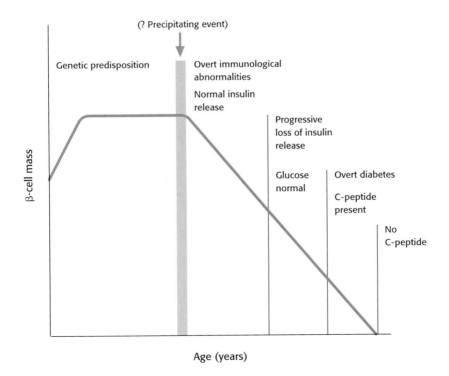

Figure 2.1 Stages in the development of IDDM.

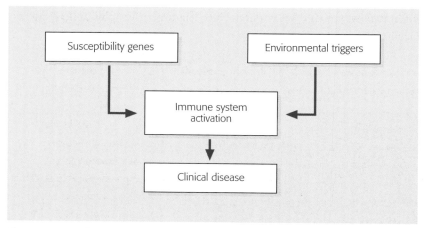

Figure 2.2 Aetiology of IDDM.

TABLE 2.1

Characteristic features of IDDM

- Insulin treatment mandatory

- Tendency to ketosis

- Onset often acute

- Onset can occur at any age, but is most common in youth

- Strong association with histocompatibility (HLA) alleles DR3 and DR4

- Autoantibodies present

- Positive family history in 10% of patients

- 50% concordance in identical twins

Pancreatic abnormalities

Pancreatic changes in IDDM are confined to the β-cells; the other cell types found in the islets of Langerhans (i.e. α-cells, δ-cells and pancreatic polypeptide cells) are unaffected. A triggering event, such as a viral infection in an individual with a genetic predisposition, provokes inappropriate humoral (mediated by B lymphocytes) and cellular (mediated by T lymphocytes and cytotoxic 'killer' cells) responses directed against the β-cells. This leads to an inflammatory reaction in which the islets are infiltrated by lymphocytes, mononuclear cells and neutrophils, referred to as insulitis (Figure 2.3).

These immune responses lead to the formation of a variety of autoantibodies (Table 2.2). Islet cell antibodies (ICA) can be detected in serum by indirect immunofluorescence (Figure 2.4). ICA are detectable

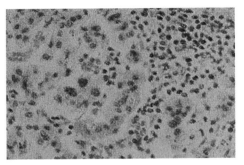

Figure 2.3 IDDM results from a progressive loss of β-cells due to chronic inflammation and destruction of the islets (insulitis) as shown in this histological section from a newly diagnosed patient.

TABLE 2.2

Autoantibodies present in IDDM

Non-specific

- Islet cell antibodies (ICA)

Specific

- Glutamic acid decarboxylase (GAD) antibodies
- Insulin antibodies
- Antibodies to tyrosine phosphatase (ICA 512)

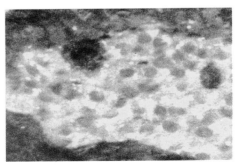

Figure 2.4 Islet cell antibodies (ICA) in patients with IDDM can be detected by indirect immunofluorescence.

11

before diabetes mellitus becomes clinically overt, but usually disappear within months of the clinical diagnosis; the reason for this is unclear. There are also three specific autoantibodies used to detect IDDM including those to insulin itself, to glutamic acid decarboxylase (GAD) and to tyrosine phosphatase (ICA 512). The use of autoantibody markers has made the prediction of future IDDM in non-diabetic subjects increasingly accurate. It has been calculated that if all three of the specific markers are positive, then the risk of susceptible individuals developing IDDM is 40–50% within 5 years.

As the autoimmune reaction progresses, the first phase of insulin secretion after food ingestion disappears and peak responses decline. However, blood glucose concentrations remain relatively normal during this phase. Symptoms of diabetes mellitus appear when the remaining β-cell mass becomes insufficient to maintain normoglycaemia. Cell loss can continue for a number of years after the diagnosis of diabetes mellitus. Indeed, the potential for autoimmune β-cell destruction persists throughout life; if, for example, pancreatic transplantation is attempted in a patient with complete loss of β-cell function, a further autoimmune response will be provoked.

Genetic factors

There is evidence for a strong genetic element in the pathogenesis of IDDM, although environmental factors also play an important role. The disease is known to cluster in families, and studies with identical twins indicate that the likelihood of both twins being affected (the concordance) is approximately 50%. The ethnic variations in prevalence may be at least partly explained by genetic factors.

A number of genetic risk factors have been reported to be associated with IDDM (Table 2.3). In particular, there is a strong association between IDDM

TABLE 2.3

Genetic risk factors associated with IDDM

- HLA-DR3 or DR4; DR3/4 heterozygous state
- HLA-DP and HLA-DQb chain polymorphism

and the class II histocompatibility (HLA) genes on chromosome 6. Approximately 95% of patients with IDDM possess the HLA-DR3 or DR4 alleles, or both; the DP and DQ alleles are also common. By contrast, the DR3 and DR4 alleles are present in only 40% of the general population. It is unclear whether HLA genes act as markers for immune response genes that promote the autoimmune reaction, or whether they contribute directly to the immune response by altering the expression of HLA glycoproteins on the β-cell surface.

Environmental factors

There is evidence to suggest that IDDM can be triggered by environmental factors in susceptible individuals.

- The incidence of IDDM is higher during the autumn and winter than during the summer.
- In children, the incidence has been reported to peak at about 5 and 12 years of age. At these ages, children would be starting or changing schools, and thus would be entering new environments. However, late onset IDDM is also recognized in patients over 65 years of age and it has been proposed that up to 15% of Caucasian NIDDM patients do, in fact, have late onset IDDM.
- Short-term changes in incidence, which can not be explained by changes in genetic susceptibility, have been reported in a number of countries.

A number of environmental factors have been proposed as possible triggers of IDDM (Table 2.4).

Viruses. Several viruses, including Coxsackie B4, mumps and rubella, have been implicated in the development of IDDM. Congenital rubella infection is the only environmental agent that has been clearly associated with IDDM.

TABLE 2.4

Environmental factors that may trigger the development of IDDM

- Viruses
- N-nitroso food additives
- Toxins

The incidence of this infection is low, however, and no other epidemiological associations between viruses and IDDM have been unequivocally identified.

N-nitroso compounds. Epidemiological studies in Iceland have shown a correlation between the incidence of IDDM and the consumption of smoked and cured mutton. Such meats contain N-nitroso compounds and it is possible that these could give rise to nitrosamines that are toxic to β-cells. Nitrosamines are structurally related to the pesticide Vacor, which has been shown to cause diabetes mellitus in humans, and to streptozotocin, which is widely used to produce experimental diabetes in animals. N-nitroso food additives could, therefore, be environmental triggers for IDDM.

Toxins. There is some evidence that breastfeeding is associated with a low incidence of IDDM. It has been suggested, therefore, that milk substitutes or commercial baby foods may contain toxins that provoke autoimmune responses in the pancreas of susceptible individuals. Similarly, cows' milk may be antigenic in individuals with a genetic predisposition to diabetes mellitus.

CHAPTER 3

What is NIDDM?

In contrast to IDDM, the pathophysiology of NIDDM is not clearly established. The principal underlying defects appear to be reduced insulin sensitivity (insulin resistance) and impaired β-cell function, which together initiate a chain of events that leads ultimately to a widespread metabolic imbalance. NIDDM often has a slow onset and therefore complications are common at the time of clinical diagnosis. The characteristic features of NIDDM are summarized in Table 3.1.

TABLE 3.1

Characteristic features of NIDDM

- Onset usually occurs in patients > 30 years of age[1]

- Onset is often insidious

- Ketosis can occur, but is uncommon

- No association with HLA genes

- No islet cell antibodies

- Positive family history in 30% of cases

- Almost 100% concordance in identical twins

- Symptoms controlled by diet and/or oral anti-hyperglycaemic drugs; insulin treatment optional (short-term treatment may be appropriate in some patients)

[1] Maturity-onset diabetes of youth (MODY) is a form of NIDDM.

Insulin resistance

The term insulin resistance indicates that the biological effect of insulin is reduced. The exact underlying cause of the insulin resistance in NIDDM is unclear. At the cellular level, insulin acts via specific receptors located within the plasma membrane. This starts a cascade of post-receptor reactions within the cell. The end result is the control of key enzymes to regulate glucose, fatty acid and amino acid metabolism within the cell (Figure 3.1). In addition, insulin controls glucose transport proteins which move glucose

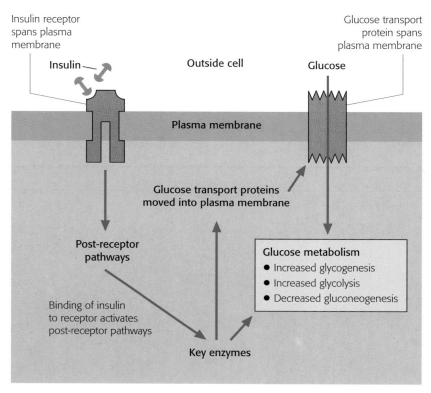

Figure 3.1 Cellular mode of action of insulin on glucose metabolism.

into the cells of muscle and fat. Insulin resistance seen in NIDDM is at the post-receptor level. The net effects of insulin resistance are seen on the liver and peripheral tissues (Figure 3.2).

β-cell failure

The exact cause of defective β-cell function in NIDDM is unknown. In NIDDM, fasting insulin concentrations correlate with fasting blood glucose levels. The relationship is that of an inverted U shape (Figure 3.3). As the fasting plasma glucose level rises, so the basal insulin rises until the glucose level is about 8 mmol/litre, when any further rise in the glucose level is associated with a decease in the basal insulin level. The basal insulin level only falls below normal in severely hyperglycaemic NIDDM patients who are nearing an insulin-requiring state.

Combination of insulin resistance and β-cell failure

It is not clear whether insulin resistance or β-cell failure is the primary defect in NIDDM, but in conceptual terms it is useful to consider both in the development of NIDDM. The insulin resistance results in compensatory hyperinsulinaemia. When β-cell function fails to compensate for increased insulin resistance, impaired glucose tolerance (IGT) arises. As β-cell function

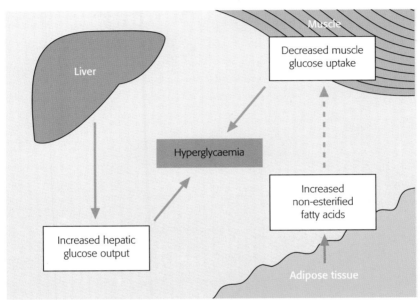

Figure 3.2 Insulin resistance and hyperglycaemia in NIDDM.

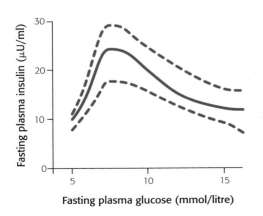

Figure 3.3 Association between fasting blood glucose and insulin concentrations in NIDDM.

continues to deteriorate, glucose tolerance falls further resulting in NIDDM and, eventually, severe β-cell failure requiring insulin therapy (Figure 3.4).

Genetic factors

Genetic factors appear to play a leading role in the pathogenesis of NIDDM. Evidence for this comes from studies of identical twins, which have shown concordance rates of almost 100%. Moreover, the prevalence of NIDDM among first degree relatives of patients with NIDDM is significantly higher than in the general population; there is a positive family history of diabetes mellitus in up to 30% of patients with NIDDM. Further evidence comes from the finding that certain ethnic groups, such as the Pima Indians of Arizona, have a high prevalence of NIDDM. In these populations, NIDDM

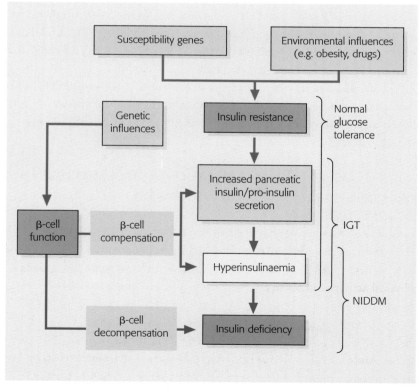

Figure 3.4 Insulin resistance and hyperinsulinaemia with impaired β-cell function leads to impaired glucose tolerance (IGT) and then NIDDM.

is often associated with obesity; this may reflect a change to a Western-style diet, with increased intakes of refined carbohydrates and fats.

In contrast to IDDM, NIDDM is not associated with specific HLA genes. There appears to be some association between NIDDM and specific alleles at the polymorphic 5'-flanking region of the insulin gene, but no specific genetic markers for NIDDM have been identified to date.

Environmental factors

The prevalence of NIDDM increases in populations where high calorie intake, limited physical activity and obesity are common. This suggests that, in addition to genetic predisposition, environmental factors play an important role in the development of this condition.

Obesity. About 65–70% of NIDDM patients are obese. Obesity leads to insulin resistance through a reduction in the number and activity of cellular insulin receptors, with a resultant decrease in glucose transport into cells and defective intracellular glucose metabolism.

The distribution of obesity is also an important risk factor for NIDDM. Individuals with a high waist:hip ratio (abdominal or central obesity) have a higher risk of developing diabetes mellitus than those with a lower waist:hip ratio.

Diet. Epidemiological evidence suggests that the incidence of NIDDM is relatively high when food is plentiful and declines during food shortages (e.g. in Europe during the two World Wars). Case-control studies have shown associations between diabetes mellitus and consumption of refined carbohydrates and fats, and diets with high energy contents. The influence of diet, however, is likely to be affected by factors such as genetic susceptibility, physical activity and obesity.

Drugs. β-blockers, corticosteroids, thiazides and loop diuretics may aggravate insulin resistance or interfere with β-cell insulin secretion. Compounded preparations of high dose β-blockers and thiazides used to treat hypertension in obese patients, with or without a family history of NIDDM, may precipitate the condition. In susceptible individuals, NIDDM often persists after the drug is withdrawn.

TABLE 3.2

Characteristics of the metabolic syndrome

- Insulin resistance
- Hyperinsulinaemia
- Central obesity
- Glucose intolerance (NIDDM or impaired glucose tolerance)
- Hypertension
- Increased levels of VLDL triglycerides
- Decreased HDL cholesterol
- Atherosclerosis

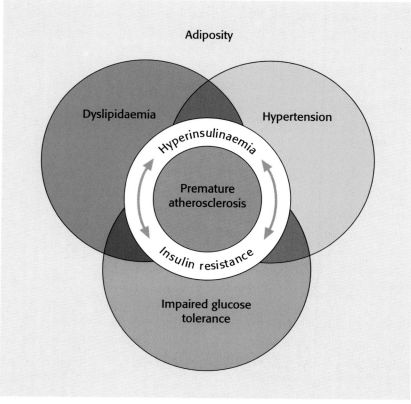

Figure 3.5 The metabolic syndrome (insulin resistance syndrome).

The metabolic syndrome

The metabolic syndrome is also known as the insulin resistance syndrome, syndrome X or Reaven's syndrome. The syndrome describes the clustering together within individuals of certain cardiovascular risk factors associated with insulin resistance and hyperinsulinaemia (Table 3.2). Whether all components of the metabolic syndrome are related to insulin resistance remains debatable, but the syndrome is associated with an increased risk of cardiovascular disease (Figure 3.5). It seems that intra-abdominal obesity causes an increase in hypertension and cardiovascular disease independently of hyperglycaemia. Hyperglycaemia causes microvascular disease and can accelerate macrovascular disease through hypertriglyceridaemia and advanced glycosylation end products (Figure 3.6).

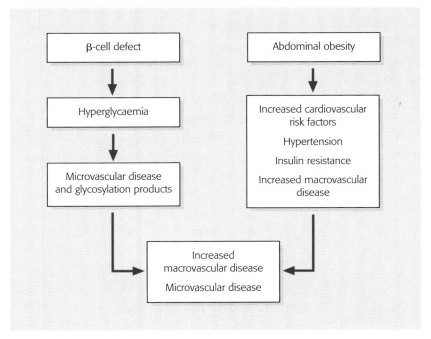

Figure 3.6 Contribution of abdominal obesity and β-cell failure to the chronic microvascular and macrovascular complications of NIDDM.

CHAPTER 4

Complications of diabetes

Diabetes mellitus can produce a variety of acute (see Chapter 9) and chronic complications (Table 4.1). Most of the morbidity and mortality associated with diabetes mellitus is, however, attributable to the chronic complications.

It is important to recognize that all diabetic patients are at risk of complications: indeed, many patients with NIDDM are asymptomatic and complications may be the presenting signs.

Microvascular complications

Microvascular complications are specific to diabetes mellitus and do not occur in non-diabetic individuals.

Diabetic retinopathy. In Western countries, diabetes mellitus is the most common cause of blindness in people aged 20–60 years. The incidence of retinopathy is related to the duration of the diabetes and the degree of glycaemic control achieved during treatment. Approximately 80–90% of patients will show some degree of retinopathy 20 years after diagnosis; 5–10% of patients with NIDDM, however, may have retinopathy at the time of diagnosis because of the insidious onset of the disease.

TABLE 4.1

Complications of diabetes

Acute
- Hypoglycaemia
- Diabetic coma

Chronic

Microvascular disorders
- Retinopathy
- Nephropathy
- Neuropathy
- Foot problems

Macrovascular disorders
- Cardiovascular disease
- Cerebrovascular disease
- Peripheral vascular disease

Diabetic retinopathy is characterized by capillary dilatation and leakage, capillary occlusion and, subsequently, new vessel formation. Capillary damage is probably related to a combination of metabolic factors associated with diabetes mellitus and haemodynamic changes, in particular an increased retinal blood flow secondary to hyperglycaemia. A number of characteristic abnormalities can be seen on fundoscopy (Table 4.2).

TABLE 4.2

Classification of diabetic retinopathy and the associated opthalmic changes

Background (simple) retinopathy

- Microaneurysms
- Haemorrhages
- Hard exudates
- (Macula not involved)

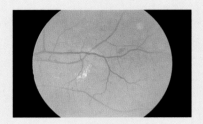

Preproliferative retinopathy

- Soft exudates (see right)
- Intra-retinal microvascular abnormalities (IRMA)
- Venous abnormalities

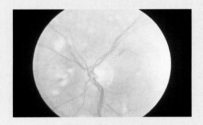

Proliferative retinopathy

- New vessel formation
- Vitreous haemorrhage
- Rubeosis iridis and secondary glaucoma may be complications

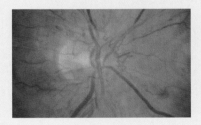

Maculopathy

- Multiple small haemorrhages around the macula (diffuse haemorrhagic maculopathy)
- Hard exudates around the macula (focal exudative maculopathy – see right)

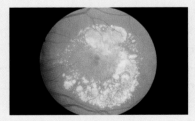

- Appearance may be normal, but vision impaired due to oedema or ischaemia (diffuse oedematous or ischaemic maculopathy)

- Microaneurysms (dot haemorrhages) appear as small, well-defined dots adjacent to vessels, may occur in clusters and sometimes regress.
- Retinal haemorrhages may be visible.
- Hard exudates, which result from capillary leakage, are waxy in appearance, with clear borders, and can occur singly, in clusters or in rings.
- Soft exudates (cotton wool spots) result from small retinal infarctions and are less clearly defined than hard exudates.
- Intra-retinal microvascular abnormalities (IRMA) precede vascular proliferation and include venous dilatation, irregularity, twisting and looping, and fibrous sheathing of the arterioles.
- New vessel formation usually occurs at the optic disc, but can also be seen peripherally at sites of vessel bifurcation. In advanced cases, it can also occur on the anterior surface of the iris (rubeosis iridis), which, if untreated, can lead to secondary glaucoma.
- Pre-retinal or vitreous haemorrhages are due to bleeding from new vessels.
- Fibrous tissue formation (retinitis proliferans) is associated with new vessel formation. This can lead to tractional retinal detachment or macular damage.

Diabetic retinopathy is classified into four types (Table 4.2). Background retinopathy occurs in a significant proportion of patients over 15–20 years of age, but can occur at any time. It may persist for several years without progressing, or occasionally may regress spontaneously. Preproliferative retinopathy leads to new vessel formation within 2 years in over 30% of patients. Proliferative retinopathy affects approximately 10% of diabetic patients, particularly those with long-standing IDDM. It is asymptomatic until vitreous haemorrhage (Figure 4.1) occurs, leading to loss of vision (advanced diabetic eye disease). If untreated, proliferative retinopathy is associated with a 50% risk of blindness within 5 years. Other features of advanced diabetic eye disease include fibrous tissue deposition and rubeosis iridis (Figure 4.1). Maculopathy mainly affects older patients with NIDDM, and may be present at the time of diagnosis.

Diabetic nephropathy develops in 30–40% of IDDM patients, two-thirds of whom will progress to end-stage renal failure (ESRF). It may also occur in

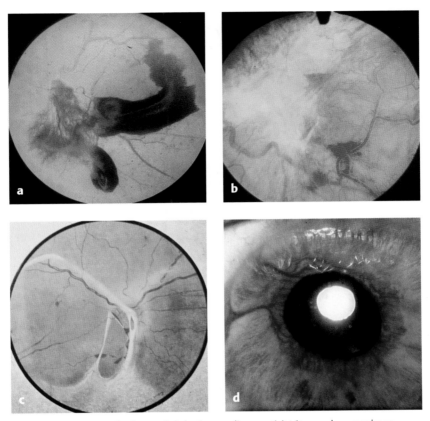

Figure 4.1 Features of advanced diabetic eye disease. (a) Vitreous haemorrhage. (b) Retinitis fibricans. (c) Traction vitreous bands. (d) Rubeosis iridis.

up to 15–20% of NIDDM patients, in 50% of whom it will progress to renal failure. Diabetic nephropathy is becoming the single most common cause of ESRF. In Europe, over 10% of those requiring dialysis or transplantation have diabetes mellitus and this figure is at least twice as high in the USA. The incidence and prevalence of diabetic nephropathy are 2–3 times greater in Asian and Afro-Caribbean patients.

The natural history of diabetic nephropathy is well defined in IDDM, but to a lesser degree in NIDDM. There are five distinct stages in the development of diabetic nephropathy in IDDM (Table 4.3).

- Early renal hypertrophy and hyperfiltration are found at diagnosis and may be partly reversed by insulin therapy.

25

TABLE 4.3

Progression of renal disease in patients with IDDM

Stage	Characteristics	Onset	Proportion progressing to next stage (%)
1	Early hypertrophy and hyperfiltration	Onset of diabetes mellitus	100
2	Microscopic renal lesions No clinical signs	2–3 years	35–40
3	Incipient nephropathy	10–15 years	80–100
4	Clinically overt nephropathy	10–30 years	75–100
5	End-stage renal failure	20–40 years	–

- Morphological glomerular lesions, without clinical disease, develop silently over many years and may be detected by renal function tests or biopsy (Figure 4.2).
- Incipient nephropathy develops in 35–40% of patients and is characterized by microalbuminuria – albumin excretion rate (AER) of 30–300 mg/24 hours (20–200 µg/minute).

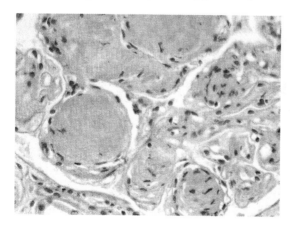

Figure 4.2 Diabetic nephropathy showing diffuse glomerulosclerosis with basement membrane thickening and areas of fibrin deposition called Kimmelstiel-Wilson nodules.

- Overt nephropathy is characterized by macroproteinuria with an AER of over 300 mg/24 hours (200 µg/minute).
- ESRF develops within 10 years of the onset of macroproteinuria.

In NIDDM, diabetic nephropathy is thought to follow a similar course, but over a shorter time scale. This is because these patients are often older and diabetes mellitus has usually been present but undiagnosed for some years.

Diabetic neuropathy may affect any part of the nervous system (cranial, peripheral, autonomic). Both somatic and autonomic neuropathies are well recognized in diabetes mellitus and often have debilitating effects. These complications can result from metabolic changes resulting in demyelination, and microvascular changes such as ischaemia. Diabetic neuropathy is a common cause of foot problems.

Chronic peripheral neuropathy affects sensory function more than motor. The appreciation of touch, pain and temperature sensation is lost, and proprioreception in the lower limbs is absent, in a 'stocking' distribution typical of a peripheral neuropathy with loss of ankle jerks and later knee jerks. The anaesthetic foot may be repeatedly traumatized leading to indolent ulceration (Figure 4.3).

Acute peripheral neuritis presents as burning foot pain, which is often worse at night and may keep the diabetic patient awake. It is associated with poor glycaemic control, but paradoxically, in some cases, it is precipitated by the institution of good control. In most patients, there is little objective evidence of neuropathy other than hyperaesthesiae (e.g. bedclothes may

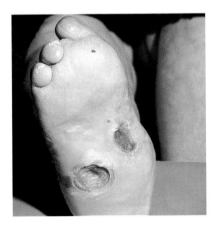

Figure 4.3 Loss of pain sensation due to peripheral neuropathy can lead to prolonged injury to the foot and consequent ulceration. Note the loss of two toes through previous amputation.

cause nocturnal pain). Continuous pain causes depression, anorexia and resultant weight loss, which in older patients may raise the suspicion of a carcinomatous neuropathy.

Mononeuropathy results in isolated palsies of either cranial or peripheral nerves; for example, IIIrd or VIth nerve palsies causing diplopia, median nerve palsy causing carpal tunnel syndrome and lateral popliteal nerve palsy causing foot drop. Occasionally, more than one nerve may be involved, giving rise to mononeuritis multiplex.

Amyotrophy is the main motor manifestation of diabetic neuropathy with painful wasting of thigh and pelvic girdle muscles (Figure 4.4). It may be the presenting feature in elderly diabetic patients. Amyotrophy may be asymmetrical and extensor plantar responses may be seen.

Autonomic neuropathy has a number of manifestations, which are listed in Table 4.4.

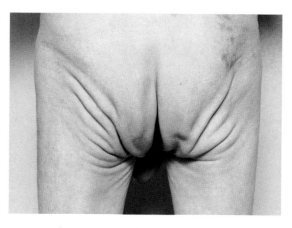

Figure 4.4 Diabetic neuropathy may present as amyotrophy, with wasting of the thigh and, as in this case, the glutei muscles.

Macrovascular complications

Macrovascular complications are not specific to diabetes mellitus and can occur in non-diabetic individuals. In diabetic patients, however, atherosclerotic vascular disease is more diffuse, and coexistent cardiac, cerebral and peripheral vascular disease is common. Macrovascular disease also arises at an earlier age than in non-diabetic individuals and affects both sexes equally.

The aetiology of the macrovascular disease in diabetes mellitus is complex. Glycaemic control plays an important role in IDDM and probably

TABLE 4.4

Abnormalities seen in autonomic neuropathy

- Impotence, which affects up to a third of diabetic men
- Loss of cardiovascular reflexes, postural hypotension, and syncope
- Constipation or diarrhoea
- Nausea and vomiting
- Urinary retention
- Abnormal pupillary reflexes
- Gustatory sweating (sweating after tasting food)

also in NIDDM. In NIDDM, however, the genetic predisposition to NIDDM itself and, particularly, the so-called metabolic syndrome or insulin resistance syndrome with hyperinsulinaemia are also involved (see Chapter 3). Hypertension and dyslipidaemia are common in such cases and it is the interplay of these cardiovascular risk factors, together with others such as cigarette smoking, that is most likely promote and enhance macrovascular disease in NIDDM patients more than in non-diabetic individuals (Table 4.5).

Cardiovascular disease is the major cause of death and hospitalization in diabetic patients. The risk of myocardial infarction or angina pectoris is 2–4 times higher among diabetic patients than in the general population, and mortality from cardiac failure and myocardial infarction is also higher. The risk of cardiovascular disease increases when any of three major risk factors – hypercholesterolaemia, diastolic hypertension and smoking – are present (Figure 4.5).

Hypertriglyceridaemia resulting from poor diabetic control also increases the risk of cardiovascular disease. These additional risks can be reduced by stopping smoking, and treatment of the hypertension and hyperlipidaemias.

Cerebrovascular disease. The incidence of cerebrovascular disease in diabetic patients is approximately 2–4 times higher than that in non-diabetic individuals.

TABLE 4.5

Relative risks for cardiovascular disease in diabetic patients compared with non-diabetic individuals, aged 35–64 years[1]

	Men	Women
Coronary heart disease	1.8	3.9
Death from coronary heart disease	2.1	4.9
Congestive heart failure	6.1	9.8
Stroke	2.8	1.9
Intermittent claudication	2.8	9.1
Total relative risk	3	4

[1]Data from the Framingham 30-year follow-up study.

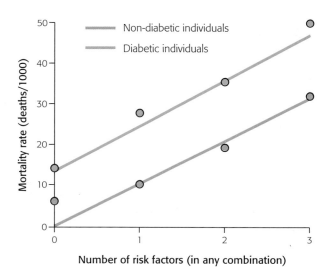

Figure 4.5 Mortality from cardiovascular disease is higher in diabetic patients than in non-diabetic individuals, and the risk increases further when major risk factors (hypercholesterolaemia, diastolic hypertension and smoking) are present. (Data from American Diabetes Association. *Diabetes Care* 1993;16 (suppl 2):573–579.)

Peripheral vascular disease. The incidence of peripheral vascular disease is increased up to six-fold in diabetes mellitus. It may present as intermittent claudication, ulceration or gangrene. Reduced or absent foot pulses, and an atrophied appearance of the foot, may also indicate impaired circulation.

Diabetic foot problems

Foot problems are a major cause of morbidity and one of the most common reasons for hospital admissions in diabetes mellitus.

The diabetic foot represents a spectrum of disorders ranging from vascular insufficiency, neuropathy and infection, to gangrene (Figure 4.6). The most important predisposing factor is neuropathy; numb feet are easily damaged (e.g. ill-fitting shoes, hot water bottles). Vascular insufficiency means that healing of even small ulcers may take months. In patients with

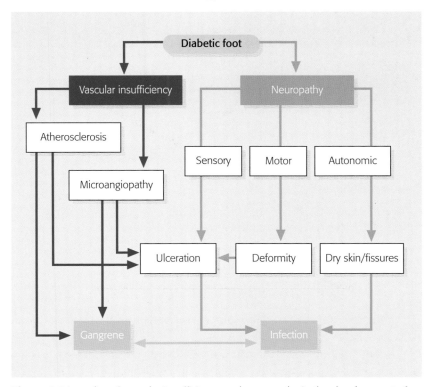

Figure 4.6 Interplay of vascular insufficiency and neuropathy in the development of infection and gangrene in the diabetic foot.

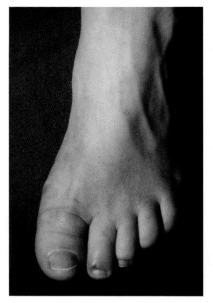 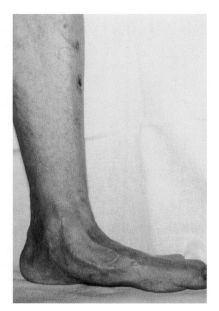

Figure 4.7 Distended superficial veins in the foot of a patient with autonomic neuropathy.

Figure 4.8 Charcot's arthropathy of mid-talar joint resulting from joint denervation and abnormal bone blood flow due to autonomic neuropathy.

autonomic neuropathy, the foot may be deceptively warm to the touch with distended superficial veins (Figure 4.7), but is very vulnerable to damage. This neuropathy together with loss of proprioreception leads to joint destruction in the lower limbs causing Charcot's athropathy (Figure 4.8).

CHAPTER 5
Diagnosis of IDDM and NIDDM

The typical clinical presentations of IDDM and NIDDM are summarized in Table 5.1. IDDM usually occurs in younger patients (< 35–40 years of age, with a peak in incidence during the teenage years), but can occur at any age. It is characterized by the 'classic' symptoms of diabetes mellitus, notably thirst and polyuria, which have a relatively sudden onset. A triggering event, such as a viral infection, may be identifiable. By contrast, NIDDM usually occurs in older patients with a progressive history of symptoms, which may extend over several years. Complications may be present; indeed, these may be the reason for consulting the doctor. NIDDM may also be an incidental finding; in population surveys, 50% of NIDDM patients are relatively asymptomatic at diagnosis.

TABLE 5.1

Clinical presentation of IDDM and NIDDM

IDDM	NIDDM
● Thirst	● Thirst
● Polyuria	● Polyuria
● Fatigue and malaise	● Fatigue and malaise
● Weight loss	● Infections (e.g. candidiasis)
● Blurred vision	● Blurred vision
● Nausea and vomiting	● Complications
● Ketoacidosis	● Incidental finding

Diabetes mellitus is usually easily diagnosed on the basis of symptoms and blood glucose concentrations (Figure 5.1). It should be noted that glycated haemoglobin values *per se* are not used for the diagnosis of diabetes mellitus.

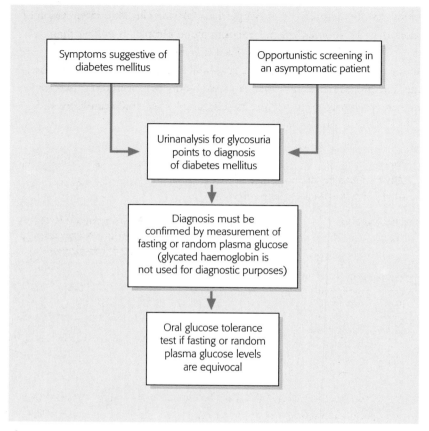

Figure 5.1 Diagnosis of diabetes mellitus.

Symptoms

The most common symptoms include:

- thirst
- polyuria (a result of excessive glucose excretion)
- weight loss (usually in IDDM, less often in NIDDM)
- pruritus vulvae or balanitis (resulting from *Candida* infection)
- blurred vision (due to osmotic lens change).

Blood glucose concentration

Glucose can be detected in the urine using simple dipstick tests; a positive result suggests the presence of diabetes mellitus, but must be confirmed by a blood test. In the presence of symptoms, a plasma glucose concentration of more than 11.1 mmol/litre in a random blood sample, or greater than 7.8 mmol/litre in a fasting sample confirms the diagnosis (Table 5.2). In the absence of symptoms, the test should be repeated. Some laboratories measure glucose concentrations in whole blood; the threshold values for diabetes mellitus in random and fasting samples are 10.0 mmol/litre and 7.0 mmol/litre, respectively.

TABLE 5.2

WHO criteria for the diagnosis of diabetes (using venous plasma glucose levels)

Classification	Fasting plasma glucose level (mmol/litre)	Plasma glucose level 2 hours after glucose load (mmol/litre)
Normal	< 6.0	< 7.8
Impaired glucose tolerance	< 7.8	7.8–11.1
Diabetes mellitus	> 7.8	> 11.1

Oral glucose tolerance test (OGTT). This test is seldom necessary, except in the few patients in whom the blood glucose test results are equivocal. The OGTT involves measuring the fasting blood glucose level, giving the subject a 75 g oral dose of glucose, and measuring the blood glucose levels again 2 hours later. A 2-hour plasma glucose concentration of 11.1 mmol/litre or above indicates diabetes mellitus; levels between 7.8 and 11.1 mmol/litre indicate impaired glucose tolerance (IGT; Figure 5.2).

Impaired glucose tolerance

IGT is a term that was introduced to differentiate individuals with slightly decreased glucose tolerance without overt diabetes from non-diabetic individuals or patients with clinical diabetes mellitus.

IGT is common, affecting about 15–20% of people aged 45–74 years in the USA and about 15% of those aged 40–65 years in the UK. IGT is not associated with the microvascular complications of diabetes mellitus (see

35

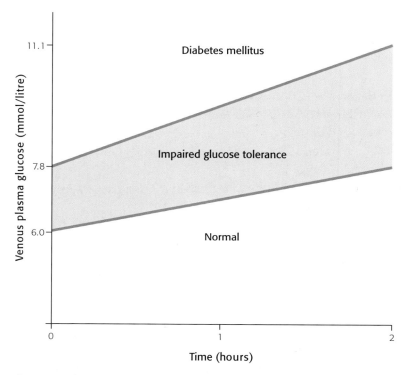

Figure 5.2 The oral glucose tolerance test is a useful diagnostic tool in patients whose blood glucose results are equivocal.

Chapter 4); it is, however, associated with an increased risk of ischaemic heart disease. About 50% of individuals with IGT revert to normal glucose tolerance within 10 years through weight loss and exercise, some 25% remain glucose intolerant and the remaining 25% develop NIDDM. Annual screening by measurement of a fasting or 2-hour plasma glucose level is recommended as follow-up for those individuals with IGT. In such individuals, risk factors for cardiovascular disease are often increased and these should also be treated.

CHAPTER 6

Treatment of IDDM

Insulin therapy has been in clinical use for about 75 years. The indications for insulin therapy can be summarized as:

- diabetic patients younger than 40–45 years, unless obese
- all diabetic patients with severe hyperglycaemic symptoms, weight loss and ketosis, irrespective of age
- older NIDDM diabetic patients not sufficiently well controlled by oral anti-hyperglycaemic drugs (see Chapter 7).

Insulin treatment

The aims of insulin treatment are:

- to prevent death from ketoacidosis
- to relieve the symptoms of uncontrolled diabetes mellitus
- to maintain blood glucose as close to normal as possible.

The Diabetic Control and Complications Trial (DCCT) has shown that glycaemic control aimed at keeping blood glucose within the normal range of 4–8 mmol/litre with a HbA_{1C} of about 7% significantly reduces the development of long-term complications (Figure 6.1; see Chapter 8). Such control should, therefore, be the aim in as many patients as possible. 'Acceptable' control, aimed at relieving symptoms without maintaining normoglycaemia, is appropriate in elderly or handicapped patients, and patients with a limited life expectancy. Good control requires careful education of the patient with respect to insulin injection technique, self-monitoring of blood glucose, and the contribution of factors such as diet, exercise and illness to insulin requirements.

Insulin preparations. Today, most IDDM patients receive human insulin preparations at diagnosis. Long-standing diabetic patients may still inject porcine or bovine preparations. Irrespective of the species of insulin, the formulation of insulin can be classified into three broad types according to their duration of action.

- Unmodified, soluble or regular insulins are short acting and last 4–6 hours.

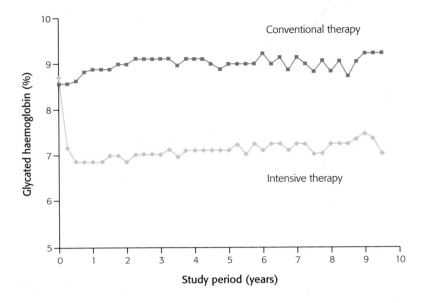

Figure 6.1 The Diabetic Control and Complications Trial (DCCT) showed that 'intensive' insulin therapy with good glycaemic control (glycated haemoglobin approximately 7.0%) resulted in fewer eye, kidney and neuropathic complications than that seen with 'conventional' insulin regimens where the glycated haemoglobin was much higher (approximately 9.0%).

- Intermediate-acting insulins (isophane type), in which action is extended by the addition of protamine or zinc, last 10–14 hours.
- Long-acting insulins (lente type), in which action is extended by addition of zinc only, last up to 24 hours.

In addition, there are so-called biphasic insulins, which are mixtures of short-acting soluble and intermediate-acting isophane type insulins in different proportions (e.g. 30/70, 50/50).

The different insulin formulations are available in vials from which the insulin is drawn up and injected subcutaneously using lightweight, pre-sterilized disposable syringes (Figure 6.2). Pen injectors, which can take refill cartridges (Figure 6.3) or be prescribed as pre-loaded pens (Figure 6.4), are being increasingly used. The usual injection sites include the upper arms,

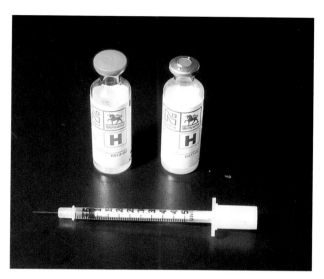

Figure 6.2 Vials of insulin with lightweight, plastic disposable syringe.

Figure 6.3 B-D Pen®/Humulin® cartridge system.

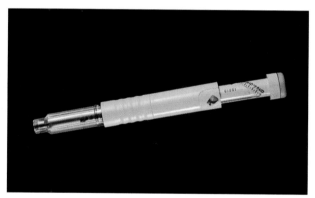

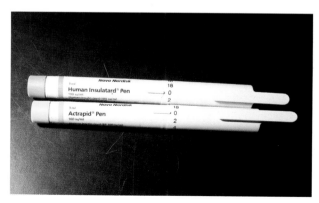

Figure 6.4 Pre-loaded disposable pens to inject Actrapid® (soluble) and Insulatard® (isophane) insulins.

thighs, buttocks or abdomen (Figure 6.5). In a few patients, insulin has been administered by continuous programmed infusion via a portable minipump, so-called continuous subcutaneous insulin infusion (CSII); these devices are, however, expensive, clumsy and prone to mechanical failure. Multiple injection regimens with basal-bolus insulin injected with a pen device are being increasingly used instead of CSII (see page 42).

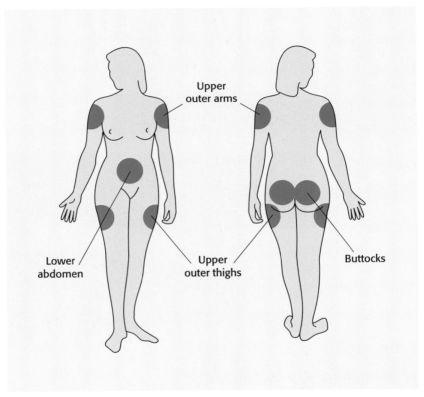

Figure 6.5 Subcutaneous insulin injection sites.

Insulin regimens are designed to mimic both the basal secretion and the postprandial surges in insulin secretion (Figure 6.6). Current insulin regimens in common use include:

- twice-daily regimens of soluble and isophane insulins, either mixed individually or using biphasic mixtures, which are injected before breakfast and before the main evening meal (Figure 6.7)

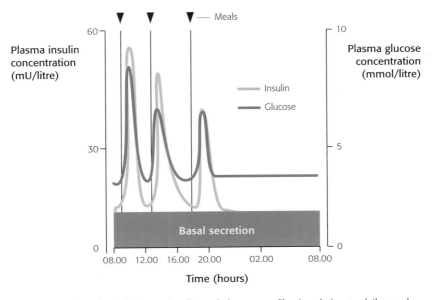

Figure 6.6 Physiological plasma insulin and glucose profiles in relation to daily meals.

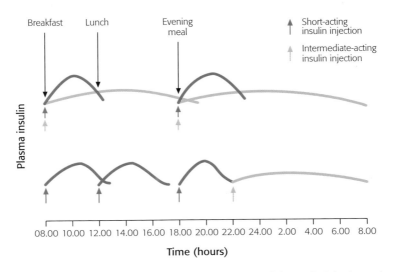

Figure 6.7 Glycaemic control can be achieved with twice-daily insulin injections of short- and intermediate-acting insulin, or by three injections of short-acting insulin at meal times followed by intermediate-acting insulin at bedtime.

- multiple injection regimens consisting of bolus injections of a soluble-type insulin (usually given with a pen injector) before breakfast, lunch and the evening meal, with a basal intermediate insulin given before bedtime (Figure 6.7).

Multiple injection regimens are preferable in younger IDDM patients who are trying to achieve the best possible glycaemic control. The twice-daily use of premixed insulin suspensions (as opposed to soluble and isophane insulins) are more convenient for older IDDM patients using twice-daily regimens.

Monitoring glycaemic control

Regular monitoring of blood glucose concentration by the patient at home is essential for good glycaemic control; if this is not possible, urine glucose measurements are better than no monitoring at all. The glycated haemoglobin level (HbA_1 or HbA_{1C}) can be measured to assess the mean blood glucose level over the previous 6–8 weeks.

Urine testing. Glucose testing (e.g. Diastix,® Diabur-Test 5000®) is now mainly used in NIDDM. The urine should be tested before breakfast and 2–3 hours after meal on 1–2 days/week. The problems encountered with urine testing for glucose include:

- imprecise results
- variable renal thresholds
- colour blindness.

Testing for ketones (e.g. Ketodiastix,® Ketostix®) is advisable for all IDDM patients, especially those with a high blood glucose level (> 12–15 mmol/litre), who are ill or vomiting for any reason, who are prone to ketoacidosis or who are pregnant. It is also advisable in children.

Blood glucose monitoring can be carried out using sticks (Figure 6.8) alone, or sticks and a meter. Sticks (e.g. BM 20–800,® Glucostix®) have the advantage that they are inexpensive and simple to use. A wide range of meters is available including computerized meters, and bleeping and talking meters for the blind. A disadvantage of meters is that they need to be checked regularly for accuracy and they can break down.

Blood glucose monitoring has the advantages that it is:

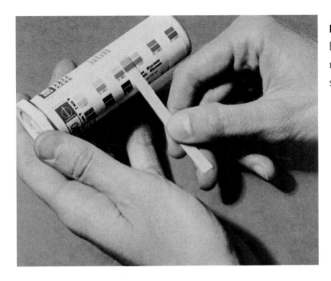

Figure 6.8 Home blood glucose monitoring using stick testing.

- more accurate than urine testing
- independent of renal threshold.

Home blood glucose monitoring is indicated in all IDDM patients and in many younger patients with NIDDM. It is especially advantageous in those aiming at tight glycaemic control, pregnant patients, and patients with difficulties in glycaemic control with variable high and low results.

Glycated haemoglobin (HbA$_1$ or HbA$_{1C}$) is formed by a non-enzymatic irreversible ketoamine linkage of glucose to the N-terminal valine of the haemoglobin chain. The higher the blood glucose level over the previous 6–8 weeks, the higher the glycated haemoglobin. There are no standards, however, for glycated haemoglobin as each laboratory has to determine its own normal range. HbA$_1$ or HbA$_{1C}$ measurements allow studies of long-term control and evaluation of different treatment regimens. For the physician, it also identifies those patients who have been 'cheating' in their home blood glucose monitoring. No assessment of overall glycaemic control in any diabetic patient, either IDDM or NIDDM, can be properly made without measurement of glycated haemoglobin. Glycated haemoglobin should be measured every 3–4 months.

CHAPTER 7

Drug treatment of NIDDM

It is now widely appreciated that NIDDM is not purely a disease of glucose control, but that the morbidity and premature mortality are closely associated with central obesity, hypertension and dyslipidaemia (increased VLDL triglycerides and decreased HDL cholesterol). It is therefore important to treat each identifiable risk factor.

The mainstay of management in NIDDM patients is appropriate dietary advice and regular exercise. However, the UK Prospective Diabetes Study (UKPDS) has recently shown that less than 20% of newly diagnosed NIDDM patients achieved good control (fasting plasma glucose ≤ 6 mmol/litre) by diet alone within 3–12 months, and longer-term studies have shown that less than 10% of NIDDM patients are controlled by dietary measures.

An approach to drug treatment in NIDDM patients in whom diet is inadequate is given in Figure 7.1. Four classes of drugs with different modes of action and different side-effect profiles are available worldwide (Table 7.1), and increasing attention is being paid to their use in step-wise

TABLE 7.1

Drugs available for glycaemic control in NIDDM and their principal mode of action

Class of drug	Mode of action
Sulphonylureas (glipizide, gliclazide, glibenclamide, chlorpropamide, tolbutamide)	Increased β-cell insulin secretion through closing ATP-sensitive potassium ion channels
Biguanides (metformin)	Decreased hepatic glucose production Increased intracellular glucose metabolism
α-glucosidase inhibitors (acarbose)	Reduction in the postprandial glucose peak by slowing gastrointestinal carbohydrate digestion
Insulin	Increased intracellular glucose oxidation and utilization Decreased hepatic glucose production

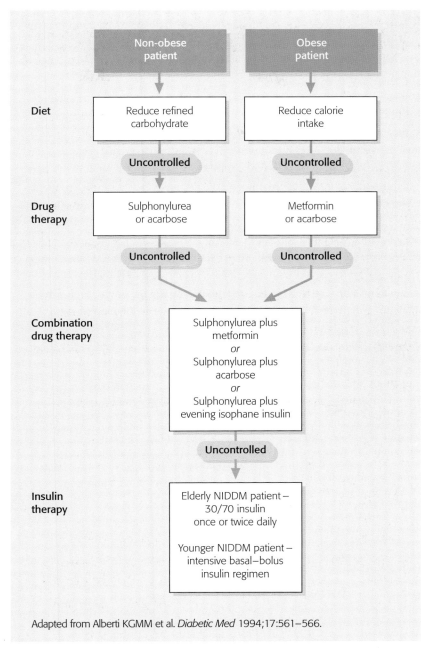

Adapted from Alberti KGMM et al. *Diabetic Med* 1994;17:561–566.

Figure 7.1 An approach to drug treatment in patients with NIDDM.

combination therapy. It is important to recognize that the best response to therapy occurs during the first few years following diagnosis. Maintenance of good glycaemic control in later years is more difficult, and often requires combinations of oral agents and occasionally insulin treatment.

Sulphonylureas

Sulphonylureas have a direct effect on the β-cells of the pancreas to promote insulin release by binding to high affinity 'sulphonylurea' receptors on the cell membrane. These drugs are rapidly absorbed from the gastrointestinal tract and transported in blood bound to plasma proteins. Their hepatic metabolism and renal excretion vary, resulting in different plasma half-lives (Table 7.2).

Indication. Sulphonylureas are indicated in non-obese NIDDM patients in whom dietary measures have failed. The use of sulphonylureas in obese individuals may result in further weight gain. Sulphonylureas may also be

TABLE 7.2

Sulphonylureas in common use

Drug	Initial dose (mg)	Dose range (mg)	Duration of action (hours)	Route of excretion
Short-acting[1]				
Tolbutamide	500	500–3000	6–10	Kidney
Intermediate-acting[1]				
Glipizide	2.5	2.5–25	15–24	Kidney 80%; bile 20%
Gliclazide	40	40–320	16–24	Kidney 70%; bile 30%
Long-acting[1]				
Chlorpropamide	100	100–500	60	Kidney
Glibenclamide	1.25	1.25–20	> 24	Kidney 50%; bile 50%

[1]Dose interval: short-acting, 2–3 times/day; intermediate-acting 1–2 times/day; long-acting, once daily.

used in combination with metformin or acarbose where monotherapy is not sufficient to control blood glucose levels.

Biguanides

Metformin is the only biguanide available for clinical use. Unlike the sulphonylureas, metformin has no direct action on the pancreatic β-cells to stimulate insulin release and its main action appears to be at a post-receptor site(s). When used as monotherapy, metformin will not induce hypoglycaemia. Metformin is absorbed from the gut, but is not bound to plasma proteins. It is not metabolized in the liver, but is excreted unchanged by the kidney, with 90% being cleared within 12 hours. The plasma half-life is short at approximately 2–3 hours. The daily maintenance dose of metformin is 0.5–3.0 g in divided doses.

Indication. Metformin is indicated for obese NIDDM patients who are not controlled by diet alone or with other oral hypoglycaemic drugs. It is preferable to the sulphonylureas because of the lack of further weight gain.

α-glucosidase inhibitors

Acarbose is the most widely available α-glucosidase inhibitor. It lowers postprandial blood glucose levels by delaying glucose absorption by competing with dietary carbohydrate for the α-glucosidase enzymes present in the microvilli of the brush border of the small intestine, which break down the oligosaccharides into monosaccharides. There is no stimulation of insulin secretion from the pancreas. As monotherapy, acarbose, like metformin, will not result in hypoglycaemia or weight gain.

Only 1–2% of acarbose is absorbed systematically. The recommended initial dose is 50 mg/day for the first 1–2 weeks, followed by 50 mg b.d. for weeks 3–4, 50 mg t.d.s. for weeks 5–6, and then titrated upwards to a dose of 100 mg t.d.s. The drug should be swallowed whole or chewed with the first mouthful of each of the three main meals.

Indication. Acarbose is indicated for NIDDM patients in whom dietary measures alone have proved insufficient or who are inadequately controlled by other anti-hyperglycaemic drugs. It is particularly useful in lowering postprandial hyperglycaemia.

Insulin

Insulin treatment is discussed in Chapter 6 in the context of the management of IDDM. However, insulin treatment may be necessary in NIDDM patients in whom inadequate glycaemic control is achieved by diet and oral anti-hyperglycaemic agents, prescribed either as monotherapy or in combination (Table 7.3). Older NIDDM patients with limited life expectancy or with severe coexistent disease are best treated with a simple regimen of either an intermediate-acting (isophane) insulin once or twice daily, or a mixture of short- and intermediate-acting insulins, to avoid the risk of hypoglycaemia. In younger NIDDM patients who are otherwise in good health, however, a more intensified insulin regimen similar to that used for IDDM patients should be given.

TABLE 7.3

Indications for insulin therapy in NIDDM

- Failure of glycaemic control with oral anti-hyperglycaemic drugs – persistent glycosuria, elevated blood glucose levels with raised glycated haemoglobin values

- Development of hyperglycaemic symptoms (e.g. thirst, polyuria, pruritus vulvae) associated with poor glycaemic control; watch for insidious onset of tiredness and malaise which may be the only complaint. Insulin restores feeling of well-being and good health

- Weight loss, often with frank hyperglycaemic symptoms, suggests insulin therapy may be required

---

Side-effects and drug interactions with oral anti-hyperglycaemic agents

The side-effects of the sulphonylureas, metformin and acarbose, together with those of insulin, are summarized in Table 7.4.

Sulphonylureas. Hypoglycaemia and weight gain are the most common side-effects of the sulphonylureas. Severe hypoglycaemia, which is a rare complication, has a mortality risk of approximately 10%. It is particularly important in the elderly in whom an erroneous diagnosis of cerebrovascular

TABLE 7.4

Side-effects of oral anti-hyperglycaemic agents in NIDDM

Side-effect	Sulphonylureas	Metformin	Acarbose	Insulin
Hypoglycaemia	+	–	–	+
Drug interaction	+	–	–	–
Hypersensitivity	+	–	–	–
Gastrointestinal upset	–	+	+	–
Lactic acidosis	–	+	–	–
Hyponatraemia	+	–	–	–
Cholestasis	+	–	–	–
Folate, vitamin B_{12} malabsorption	–	+	–	–
Hyperinsulinaemia	+	–	–	+
Weight gain	+	–	–	+

accident, transient ischaemic attack or even dementia may be made. A diagnosis of hypoglycaemia should be considered in any diabetic patient treated with a sulphonylurea who develops signs of altered behaviour.

The action of the sulphonylureas may be prolonged in patients with liver and renal impairment. Most sulphonylureas, except chlorpropamide, are metabolized in the liver before being excreted by the kidney and, in renal and liver impairment, the drug may accumulate. Gliclazide, however, can be useful in patients with renal impairment as less than 5% of the drug is excreted unaltered in the urine, although tolbutamide and glipizide, which have inactive metabolites may also be used.

Therapy with sulphonylureas should be initiated with low doses and increased slowly at 4–7-day intervals; rarely, a patient may be exquisitely sensitive and develop severe hypoglycaemia. Glibenclamide and chlorpropamide should be used with caution in the elderly, because they are more likely to cause hypoglycaemia than the other sulphonylureas.

TABLE 7.5

Important drug reactions with sulphonylureas

Decreased anti-hyperglycaemic effect	Increased anti-hyperglycaemic effect	'Blunt' response to hypoglycaemia
• Frusemide (not bumetanide)	• Salicylates	• β-blockers
	• Warfarin	• Clonidine
• Thiazides	• Mono-amine oxidase inhibitors	• Reserpine
• Oral contraceptives		• Guanethidine
• Corticosteroids	• Barbiturates	
• Phenytoin	• Fibrates	
• Rifampicin	• Alcohol	

Drugs that antagonize and potentiate the anti-hyperglycaemic effect of sulphonylureas, as well as drugs that mask the awareness of impending hypoglycaemia are summarized in Table 7.5.

Metformin. Gastrointestinal side-effects, with anorexia, abdominal discomfort, nausea, diarrhoea and a metallic taste in the mouth, may occur with metformin. If the dose of metformin is started at 0.5 g b.d. and built up slowly, and the tablets are taken after meals, only about 2–5% of patients are intolerant of the drug.

Lactic acidosis due to the biguanide phenformin was well recognized, but does not occur with metformin if the prescribing recommendations are adhered to (i.e. exclusion of patients with liver and renal disease, withdrawal of drug in patients with a severe acute illness which can cause hypoxia, especially respiratory or cardiac failure). Age *per se* is not a contraindication to metformin provided that renal function is satisfactory, with a serum creatinine level below 120 μmol/litre in patients aged 65 years or less and below 140 μmol/litre in those over 65 years of age.

Acarbose is generally well tolerated, but the presence of undigested carbohydrate in the gastrointestinal tract may lead to an increase in gas formation as a result of fermentation in the bowel, producing flatulence, abdominal discomfort and diarrhoea. Many of these symptoms will settle or disappear with continued treatment.

In earlier USA trials, about 4% of patients receiving acarbose in doses of up to 300 mg t.d.s. showed a mild rise in liver transaminases. This effect was not seen in similar European trials. At present, however, monitoring of serum hepatic transaminases is recommended in those patients receiving the maximum dose of 200 mg t.d.s.

Step-wise and combination drug therapy for treatment of NIDDM

The different modes of action of the various oral agents make it feasible to combine them with each other and/or insulin to provide an increasing number of options for the treatment of NIDDM patients. Figure 7.1 shows a treatment outline for NIDDM .

Patients with mild-to-moderate hyperglycaemia, that is inadequately controlled by diet and a modest increase in physical activity, can be treated with metformin or acarbose. Neither metformin nor acarbose would cause weight gain, and both may lower postprandial triglyceride levels. With more severe hyperglycaemia, with a decrease in insulin action and fall in insulin secretion, sulphonylureas are more appropriate because they increase insulin secretion. Eventually, when the sulphonylureas are less effective, combination therapy with metformin and/or acarbose would be appropriate to restore glycaemic control. As the insulin deficiency increases, an isophane insulin could be given at bedtime to control fasting hyperglycaemia with continuation of the oral agents during the day. Finally, when β-cell failure is complete and insulin secretion severely impaired, twice-daily or multiple daily insulin injections are necessary.

CHAPTER 8

Management of the long-term complications of diabetes

The long-term complications of diabetes mellitus are a major cause of morbidity and mortality. They can also substantially impair the patient's quality of life and be the cause of frequent hospitalization. Long-term complications are, therefore, an important aspect of the overall management of the diabetic patient.

The Diabetes Control and Complications Trial (DCCT) has shown that the level of glycated haemoglobin (HbA$_{IC}$) provides a means of estimating the likelihood that microvascular disease will occur and progress (Table 8.1 and Figure 8.1). These data as yet only apply to IDDM, but are relevant in NIDDM since hyperglycaemia itself is the cause of these complications. In general, intensive insulin therapy with normalization of the glycated haemoglobin will reduce the risk of retinopathy, nephropathy and neuropathy. Control of associated hypertension is also important in preventing the progression of retinopathy and nephropathy.

TABLE 8.1

Reduction of risk of retinopathy, nephropathy and neuropathy in IDDM by near normoglycaemic control (reduction of HbA$_{1C}$ from 9.0% to 7.1%)[1]

	Risk reduction (%)	
	Primary prevention	Secondary intervention
Retinopathy		
Laser treatment	76	56
Nephropathy		
Urinary albumin excretion rate > 300 mg/24 hours (> 200 μg/minute)	34	56
Neuropathy		
Clinical symptoms	69	57

[1]Data from Diabetes Control and Complications Trial. *N Engl J Med* 1993;329:977–986.

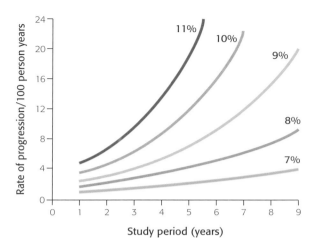

Figure 8.1 Data from the Diabetes Control and Complications Trial have clearly demonstrated that a decrease in the mean glycated haemoglobin (HbA$_{1C}$) levels slows the rate of progression of diabetic retinopathy in IDDM patients.

Management of diabetic retinopathy

Diabetic retinopathy is treatable if detected early, and regular screening is therefore essential. Visual acuity should be measured annually by means of a Snellen chart; the chart should be viewed through a pinhole to correct minor refractive abnormalities if visual acuity is reduced. The fundus should be examined with the pupils dilated (e.g. with tropicamide, 0.5–1%). The patient should be referred to an ophthalmologist if signs of preproliferative or proliferative retinopathy, or maculopathy are present and considered for photocoagulation therapy by argon laser. Patients with background retinopathy should be reviewed every 6–12 months.

Photocoagulation therapy by argon laser (Figure 8.2) is performed under topical anaesthesia. Short pulses of laser energy are used to destroy large areas of retina, thus reducing the stimulus to new vessel formation (Figure 8.3); usually 2000–3000 pulses are delivered to each eye. Laser therapy is successful in up to 90% of cases of preproliferative and proliferative retinopathy, and in 60% of cases of maculopathy. Patients with advanced diabetic eye disease – vitreous haemorrhage, fibrovascular membrane formation or traction retinal detachment – may benefit from vitrectomy.

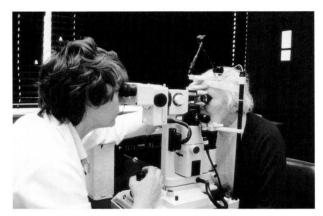

Figure 8.2 Diabetic retinopathy can be treated by photocoagulation using an argon laser.

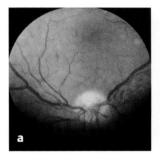
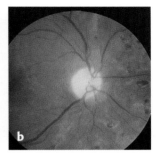

Figure 8.3 Photocoagulation destroys ischaemic areas of retina thus reducing the stimulus to new vessel formation produced by ischaemic tissue. (**a**) Before treatment. (**b**) After treatment.

This is a surgical technique in which the opaque vitreous is removed, the membranes cut, new blood vessels cauterized and the underlying ischaemic retina destroyed by intra-ocular laser ablation.

Management of diabetic nephropathy

Urine should be tested annually for microalbuminuria which is a marker of the development of more progressive renal disease. Gross protein excretion can be measured by a simple dipstick technique (Albustix). If proteinuria is present, a midstream urine sample should be analysed; a negative result in the presence of proteinuria strongly indicates diabetic nephropathy and necessitates referral. A strategy for screening for microalbuminuria is shown in Figure 8.4.

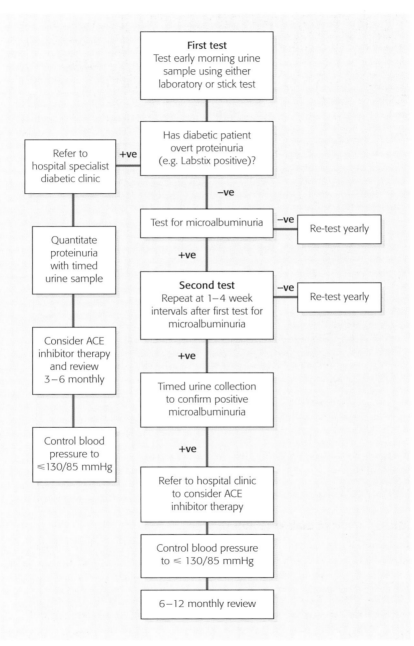

Figure 8.4 Screening strategy for microalbuminuria in family practice.

Initial management of diabetic nephropathy includes administration of an angiotensin-converting enzyme (ACE) inhibitor and control of hypertension (Table 8.2). If a significant reduction in renal function occurs, a low protein diet may be introduced which may help to delay progression. If renal function deteriorates and dialysis is required, chronic ambulatory peritoneal dialysis (CAPD) is the treatment of choice. An advantage of CAPD is that insulin can be administered with the dialysis fluid, allowing the patient to maintain good glycaemic control. Chronic haemodialysis is less suitable for diabetic patients because peripheral vascular disease and coronary heart disease are often present, and marked fluid shifts can occur. Renal transplantation has been shown to be an effective treatment in diabetic patients, although the overall benefits are less than in the non-diabetic population.

TABLE 8.2

Treatment of diabetic nephropathy

Normal urinary albumin excretion rate of ≤30 mg/24 hours (≤20 μg/minute)
- Maintain near normoglycaemic control – glycated haemoglobin (HbA_{1C}) ≤7.0%
- Maintain blood pressure ≤130/85 mmHg

Microalbuminuria – normotensive
- Maintain near normoglycaemic control – HbA_{1C} ≤ 7.0%
- Maintain blood pressure ≤130/85 mmHg
- Treat with angiotensin-converting enzyme (ACE) inhibitor

Microalbuminuria – hypertensive
- Maintain HbA_{1C} ≤ 7.0%
- Reduce blood pressure to ≤130/85 mmHg with ACE inhibitor as part of anti-hypertensive regimen

Proteinuria
- Aggressive anti-hypertensive therapy to achieve blood pressure ≤130/85mmHg
- Treat with ACE inhibitor
- Low protein diet
- Glycaemic control is of value, but to an unknown extent; an HbA_{1C} of 7.0–8.0% is acceptable

TABLE 8.3

Criteria for starting pharmacological anti-hypertensive treatment in diabetic patients

IDDM

- Younger patients with blood pressure persistently above 140/90 mmHg
- Microalbuminuria, irrespective of blood pressure

NIDDM

- Blood pressure above 135/85 mmHg, plus complications such as microalbuminuria or proteinuria, or other evidence of end-organ damage
- Blood pressures persistently above 140/90 mmHg

Management of hypertension

Hypertension is common in diabetic patients, and significantly increases the risk of progression of renal disease. Monitoring and effective control of blood pressure are, therefore, an important aspect of diabetes management. Treatment should be started at lower blood pressure levels and should be more aggressive than in non-diabetic patients. The criteria for starting pharmacological treatment are summarized in Table 8.3. Treatment should aim to achieve a diastolic blood pressure below 85 mmHg, although a lower target may be appropriate in younger IDDM patients.

When choosing an anti-hypertensive agent, drugs such as β-blockers and thiazides should be avoided, as they may reduce insulin sensitivity and aggravate dyslipidaemia, which is often seen in IDDM and, especially, NIDDM patients. ACE inhibitors, calcium channel blockers and α_1-blockers are preferable (Table 8.4).

ACE inhibitors. There is evidence that ACE inhibitors have a number of beneficial effects in diabetic patients. In clinical trials, these agents have been shown to:

- reduce urinary albumin excretion rates
- delay the development of gross proteinuria in patients with microalbuminuria (Figure 8.5)
- reduce the risk of death, dialysis or renal transplantation (Figure 8.6).

ACE inhibitors may also reduce insulin resistance, and have no adverse

57

effects on lipid or carbohydrate metabolism. Thus, their use as first-line anti-hypertensive therapy in diabetic patients, as well as their use in normotensive microalbuminuric diabetic patients, is becoming widely accepted.

TABLE 8.4

Effect of anti-hypertensive agents on insulin sensitivity and plasma lipid levels

Drug	Insulin effect	Plasma		
		Cholesterol	Triglyceride	HDL cholesterol
Thiazides	↓	↑	↑	➡
β-blockers	↓	➡	↑	↓
Angiotensin-converting enzyme (ACE) inhibitors	↑ (?)	➡	➡	➡
Calcium channel blocker	➡	➡	➡	➡
α_1-blockers	↑	↓	➡	↑

↑ increase   ➡ no change   ↓ decrease

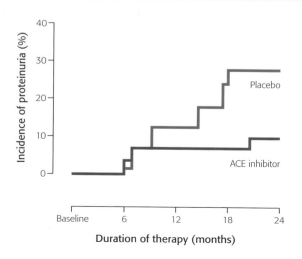

Figure 8.5

Angiotensin-converting enzyme (ACE) inhibitors have been shown to delay the development of proteinuria in patients with microalbuminuria by 70%. (Data from Viberti G et al. *JAMA* 1994;271:275–279.)

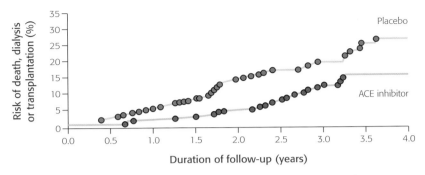

Figure 8.6 Angiotensin-converting enzyme (ACE) inhibitors have been shown to reduce the risk of death, dialysis or transplantation in patients with diabetic nephropathy by 50%. (Data from Lewis EJ et al. *N Engl J Med* 1993;329:1456–1462.)

If ACE inhibitors cannot be used or are inadequate as monotherapy to control the hypertension, and/or the proteinuria, calcium channel blockers such as verapamil can be introduced.

Management of diabetic neuropathy

Screening. Diabetic peripheral neuropathy may be identified from physical signs and symptoms, and by quantitative measurements of vibration perception threshold (VPT) using a biothesiometer, also known as neurometer. The VPT is usually measured at the first toe with the probe balanced on the pulp of the toe. A mean of three readings is used to derive a value for each foot. The VPT can be a useful predictor of foot ulceration in diabetic patients:

- a VPT of less than 15 volts represents little or no risk of foot ulceration
- a VPT of 15–25 volts represents an intermediate risk
- a VPT of more than 25 volts represents a high risk.

Chronic sensorimotor neuropathy with numb feet does not respond well to any known treatment and preventive foot care with regular supervision by a chiropodist or a podiatrist is important.

Acute peripheral neuritis improves slowly with good glycaemic control and is prevented by maintaining near normal blood glucose levels. In NIDDM patients, temporary use of insulin may be indicated until the symptoms of the neuritis settle. Drug treatment for painful neuritis is variable in its effect. Analgesics are often tried initially, and carbazepine and tricyclic antidepressants such as amitriptyline are each effective in about 30% of cases.

Diabetic amyotrophy requires intensive physiotherapy and often it takes 9–12 months for the muscle power to return to near normal.

Autonomic neuropathy. A number of simple non-invasive tests based on cardiovascular reflex can be used to identify autonomic neuropathy (Table 8.5). The various symptom complexes seen in autonomic neuropathy can only be managed in a symptomatic manner (Table 8.6) as there are no curative remedies.

Management of foot problems

The most important aspect of diabetic foot management is the education of the patient in the basic principles of good foot care (Table 8.7). The feet of a diabetic patient should be examined regularly and, if a foot

TABLE 8.5

Non-invasive tests for autonomic neuropathy

Heart rate responses
- Valsalva's manoeuvre
- Heart rate variation
- Response to standing

Blood pressure responses
- Postural fall in blood pressure
- Response to sustained hand grip

TABLE 8.7

Guide-lines for foot care in diabetic patients

- Keep feet clean. Wash in warm, not hot, water
- Use simple lotions to prevent dry, cracked skin
- Seek advice from a chiropodist on foot care
- Feet should be measured before buying shoes
- Feet should be examined regularly at family practice or hospital clinic
- Report any foot problem to nurse, chiropodist or doctor
- Avoid smoking and self-treating foot problems, and take care when walking barefoot

TABLE 8.6

Treatment for symptom complexes seen in diabetic autonomic neuropathy

Symptom	Treatment	Comment
Postural hypotension	Tilt bed at night Fludrocortisone	Antigravity suit and elastic tights are not currently used
Excessive sweating	Propantheline Poldine	These drugs may worsen gastric or bladder atony
Gastric stasis	Metoclopramide Domperidone Cisapride Erythromycin	If drugs ineffective, surgical drainage may be considered in exceptional cases
Diabetic diarrhoea	Codeine or co-phenotrope Tetracyclines α-adrenergic agonists (e.g. clonidine)	Difficult to guarantee effective therapy Spontaneous remissions
Constipation	Domperidone Metoclopramide	
Impotence	Implantable penile prostheses Vacuum constriction (non-invasive) devices Self-injection with papaverine into penis	Hormone therapy ineffective
Bladder dysfunction	Regular voiding Antibiotics for infection Catheterize Carbochol or distigmine	If drugs ineffective, consider bladder neck resection
Oedema	Ephedrine	
Hypoglycaemic unawareness	Self-monitoring of blood glucose Less stringent control	Relative(s) should be instructed in the use of glucagon
Cardiorespiratory arrest ('sudden death')	Close monitoring during 'at risk' situations (e.g. anaesthesia, chest infections)	Avoid drugs which depress respiration (e.g. opiates, hypnotics)

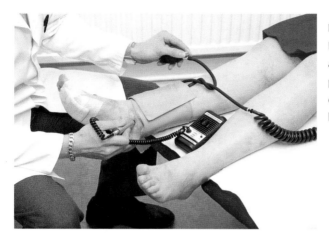

Figure 8.7
Doppler ultrasound assessment of peripheral pulses to calculate the ankle: brachial index.

problem is suspected, further tests can be arranged. These involve assessment of possible neuropathic and vascular abnormalities (see Chapter 4). Peripheral sensory function can be assessed by clinical testing of sensation and reflexes, backed by VPT measurement.

The circulation to the foot can be assessed by palpation of the foot pulses. This is, however, often difficult and Doppler ultrasound may be necessary (Figure 8.7). Reduced blood flow is indicated by an abnormal ratio between the dorsalis pedis and brachial systolic pressures, which is expressed as the ankle: brachial index (ABI). The ABI is normally over 0.9. An ABI of 0.5–0.8 is seen in intermittent claudication and an ABI of less than 0.3 in patients with pain at rest. In such cases, the patient should be referred to a vascular surgeon for urgent ateriography. Arterial surgery or angioplasty may be possible, but amputation is often required if gangrene is present.

Management of macrovascular disease

The treatment of macrovascular disease in diabetes mellitus is the same as in the general population; for example:

- thrombolytic therapy in acute myocardial infarction, even if proliferative retinopathy is present
- coronary artery bypass grafting for coronary artery disease (angina)
- angioplasty and bypass grafting in peripheral vascular disease (intermittent claudication)
- carotid endorectomy in transient cerebral ischaemic attacks.

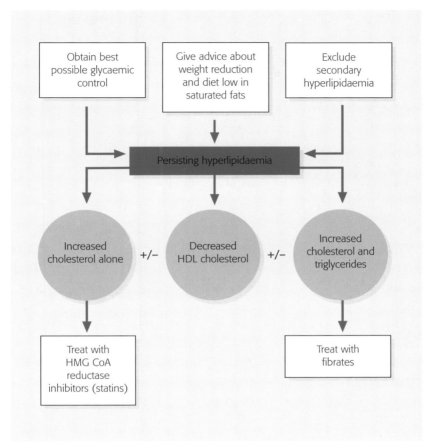

Figure 8.8 Management of dyslipidaemia in diabetes mellitus.

In clinical practice, intervention techniques for diabetic macrovascular disease are often disappointing because of the severity and widespread nature of the disease. Prevention is felt to be the best method of approaching the problem, but in NIDDM especially, the disease may be diagnosed late after years of occult glucose intolerance in middle-aged individuals who already have extensive macrovascular disease at presentation.

Dyslipidaemia
As yet, there are no trial data to indicate that lowering lipid levels will reduce the risk of cardiovascular disease in diabetic patients. However, as the

TABLE 8.8

Recommendations of the European Diabetes Policy Group for lipid control in diabetes mellitus

	Good	Borderline	Poor
Total cholesterol	< 5.2 mmol/litre (< 200 mg/dl)	< 6.5 mmol/litre (< 250 mg/dl)	> 6.5 mmol/litre (> 250 mg/dl)
HDL cholesterol	> 1.1 mmol/litre (> 40 mg/dl)	⩾0.9 mmol/litre (⩾35 mg/dl)	< 0.9 mmol/litre (< 35 mg/dl)
Fasting triglycerides	< 1.7 mmol/litre (< 150 mg/dl)	< 2.2 mmol/litre (< 200 mg/dl)	> 2.2 mmol/litre (> 200 mg/dl)

incidence of atherosclerotic vascular problems is high in both IDDM and NIDDM, it is reasonable to control any hyperlipidaemia (Table 8.8).

The treatment of dyslipidaemia in diabetes mellitus is outlined in Figure 8.8. It is important to achieve the best glycaemic control possible, as this will often improve the elevated triglyceride and lowered HDL levels. Appropriate dietary advice to reduce weight when appropriate and reduce the intake of highly saturated fats should be stressed. It is also important to exclude causes of secondary hyperlipidaemia, especially primary hypothyroidism causing hypercholesterolaemia and excessive alcohol abuse giving rise to hypertriglyceridaemia.

CHAPTER 9

Treatment of hypoglycaemia and ketoacidosis

Hypoglycaemia

Hypoglycaemia, possibly leading to coma, can occur in both IDDM and NIDDM patients. In insulin-treated patients, it can be due to insulin overdose, excessive exercise or inadequate carbohydrate intake; it can also occur in patients treated with sulphonylureas, particularly elderly patients, those with hepatic or renal disease, and those receiving potentiating drugs such as aspirin, warfarin or fibrates.

Hypoglycaemia is common. Approximately 30% of young insulin-treated patients experience a hypoglycaemic coma at some time during their lives, and the annual incidence is about 10%; recurrent comas occur in about 3% of patients. Hypoglycaemic coma is a potentially fatal complication, accounting for 3–4% of diabetes-related deaths.

Clinical features of hypoglycaemia. A plasma glucose level of less than 3 mmol/litre confirms a diagnosis of hypoglycaemia. The body's response to hypoglycaemia is to activate counter-regulatory mechanisms via the autonomic nervous system in an attempt to correct the plasma glucose. If the blood sugar continues to fall, the lack of effective glucose in the central nervous system gives rise to so-called neuroglycopenia (Figure 9.1). The clinical features of hypoglycaemia are therefore related to both adrenergic symptoms and neuroglycopenia (Table 9.1). In older patients (> 60 years), the presenting symptoms may be impaired consciousness or abnormal behaviour, which may be mistaken for a manifestation of cerebrovascular disease.

Management of hypoglycaemia. Insulin-treated patients who are conscious and able to swallow should be given oral carbohydrates (e.g. chocolate or sugary drinks). Unconscious patients should receive 50% dextrose as an intravenous bolus of 20–50 ml and, if hospitalization is required, an infusion of 10–20% dextrose to maintain the blood glucose level between 6 and 10 mmol/litre. Intramuscular or intravenous glucagon, 1 mg, may also be given, but if the hypoglycaemia has been precipitated by or is associated

65

with excess alcohol intake, glucagon may be ineffective as alcohol blocks the action of glucagon to break glycogen down into glucose. Patients who are being treated with sulphonylureas should be hospitalized even after apparent recovery, because these drugs have long half-lives and the hypoglycaemia can

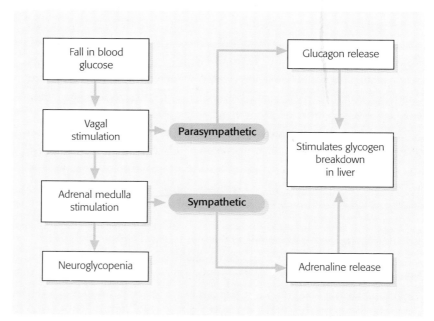

Figure 9.1 A number of counter-regulatory mechanisms are activated in response to hypoglycaemia.

TABLE 9.1

Clinical features of hypoglycaemia

Adrenergic symptoms	Neuroglycopenia
• Tachycardia	• Faintness
• Palpitations	• Feeling of hunger
• Tremor	• Headache
• Anxiety	• Abnormal behaviour
• Sweating	• Altered consciousness
	• Eventually, coma

therefore recur; in these patients, it may be necessary to continue the dextrose infusion for up to 3–5 days.

An occasional finding in patients with insulin-induced hypoglycaemia is the 'Somogyi effect', which is a combination of nocturnal hypoglycaemia and fasting hyperglycaemia. This has traditionally been believed to be due to an exaggerated counter-regulatory secretion of hormones such as glucagon, which leads to 'rebound' hyperglycaemia. It appears, however, that the effect is due to inappropriate insulin levels during the night (e.g. after an injection of long-acting insulin at bedtime). Thus, the Somogyi effect can be avoided by giving insulin in divided doses, with careful attention to the timing of each injection.

Patients with diabetic autonomic neuropathy or tightly regulated blood glucose levels may be unaware of hypoglycaemia as a result of a dampened autonomic nervous system response. These patients are, therefore, at increased risk of coma and seizures, and may need to maintain their blood glucose at a higher than ideal level.

Diabetic ketoacidosis (diabetic coma)

Despite increasing knowledge and newer technologies, the incidence of diabetic ketoacidosis is rising both throughout Europe and in the USA, with a mortality rate of up 5%.

Intercurrent illness, such as infection which is identifiable in 30–40% of episodes of diabetic ketoacidosis, may precipitate acute metabolic decompensation in diabetic patients, especially those with IDDM. A combination of an inadequate insulin supply to meet the stress situation, the secretion of catabolic hormones (catecholamines, cortisol, glucagon), together with inadequate food intake and vomiting, gives rise to hyperglycaemia and dehydration, and a metabolic acidosis (Table 9.2 and Figure 9.2). Typical fluid and electrolyte losses in diabetic ketoacidosis are listed in Table 9.3. Other biochemical findings may include:

- plasma glucose – 40 mmol/litre (720 mg/dl)
- plasma bicarbonate – 6 mmol/litre
- arterial pH – 7.12 (arterial blood H^+ – 76 mmol/litre).

The signs and symptoms of diabetic ketoacidosis are summarized in Table 9.4. Hypothermia may occur, even in the presence of infection, and may be related to hypovolaemia or acidosis-induced peripheral vasodilatation. An

67

TABLE 9.2

Factors precipitating diabetic ketoacidosis

- Infection
- Omission or reduction in insulin dose
- Acute medical or surgical illness (e.g. myocardial infarction, appendicitis)
- Emotional upsets especially in adolescence
- Menstruation
- Pregnancy ketosis
- Rare syndromes of insulin resistance

TABLE 9.3

Typical fluid and electrolyte losses in diabetic ketoacidosis

● Water	5–10 litres
● Sodium	400–700 mmol
● Chloride	300–600 mmol
● Potassium	≥ 300–700 mmol
● Magnesium	30–60 mmol
● Phosphate	50–100 mmol
● Calcium	50–100 mmol
● Alkali	300–500 mmol

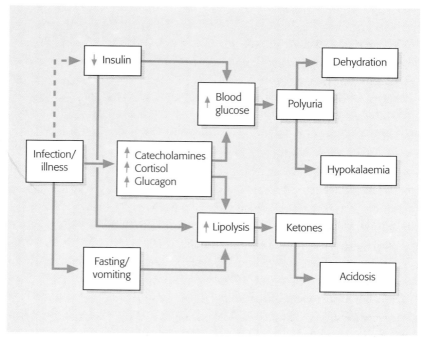

Figure 9.2 Pathogenesis of diabetic ketoacidosis.

TABLE 9.4

Clinical features of diabetic ketoacidosis

These symptoms and signs require immediate medical intervention. Insulin should never be stopped except on the instructions of a specialist.

Hyperglycaemia	Acidosis
● Dehydration	● Air hunger (Kussmaul's respiration)
● Tachycardia	● Acetone on breath
● Hypotension	● Abdominal pain
● Clouding of consciousness	● Vomiting

plus

● Features related to precipitating factors (e.g. sepsis)

elevated white blood count may be due to the acidosis *per se* and does not necessarily indicate that infection is present.

Management of diabetic ketoacidosis. Diabetic ketoacidosis is a medical emergency requiring urgent hospital admission for immediate and aggressive management. The principles of management are:

- replacement of fluid and electrolytes with intravenous saline and dextrose solutions
- a constant intravenous infusion of a soluble insulin at a rate of 6–8 units/hour
- replacement of potassium intravenously
- bicarbonate, in controlled amounts of 50–100 mmol over 1 hour in severe cases (e.g. to relieve the distress of Kussmaul's respiration)
- a prophylactic regimen of heparin in a dose of 5000 units s.c. 6-hourly if osmolality is very high (> 340 mosmol/kg)
- treat underlying cause (e.g. broad-spectrum antibiotic therapy for suspected infection while results of blood cultures, throat swabs, midstream specimen of urine and sputum are awaited).

Intravenous therapy is stopped and subcutaneous insulin reinstated when the episode of ketoacidosis is resolved, and the patient is able to eat and drink normally.

Hyperosmolar non-ketotic coma

Hyperosmolar non-ketotic coma (HONK) is a form of diabetic coma seen in older patients. It is often seen at diagnosis in previously unrecognized patients, 50% of whom may be subsequently controlled without insulin therapy. The clinical features of HONK are summarized in Table 9.5.

A diagnosis of HONK should be considered in any elderly patient who is drowsy or unconscious, and severely dehydrated, but not hyperventilating. Impaired cerebral perfusion may give rise to focal neurological signs and a cerebrovascular accident may be suspected. It is essential to test for glycosuria, hyperglycaemia and, where necessary, to measure plasma urea and electrolytes to confirm HONK. Hospital treatment is necessary and the principles of management are the same as for diabetic ketoacidosis.

TABLE 9.5

Clinical features of hyperosmolar non-ketotic coma (HONK)

- Severe hyperglycaemia – plasma glucose > 50 mmol/litre (900 mg/dl)
- Severe dehydration and hyperosmolality (> 340 mosmol/kg)
- No ketoacidosis (bicarbonate >18 mmol/litre)
- Multiple precipitating factors (e.g. thiazide or loop diuretics, excessive sugary drinks for thirst, infection, impaired renal function)

The plasma osmolality is calculated from the following formula where plasma concentrations are in mmol/litre:

$$\text{Osmolality (mosmol/kg)} = 2\,(Na^+ + K^+) + \text{urea} + \text{glucose}$$

For example:

	plasma glucose	= 60 mmol/litre,
	Na^+	= 158 mmol/litre,
	K^+	= 5.0 mmol/litre,
	urea	= 20 mmol/litre,

then: osmolality $= 2\,(158 + 5) + 20 + 60 = 406$ mosmol/kg

CHAPTER 10
Diabetes and the skin

Diabetes mellitus can affect the skin in many ways.

- Microangiopathic, atherosclerotic and neuropathic abnormalities are implicated in diabetic foot lesions (see page 31).
- Bacterial and fungal infections of the skin and mucous membranes are more common.
- Xanthomata may occur as a result of hyperlipidaemia associated with diabetes mellitus (see pages 63–64).
- Granuloma annulare, though not specific for diabetes, is more often seen in diabetes mellitus. It is a chronic skin eruption that usually affects the hands and feet, and consists of smooth, firm, flesh-coloured papules arranged in a ring around a central area of unaffected skin (Figure 10.1).

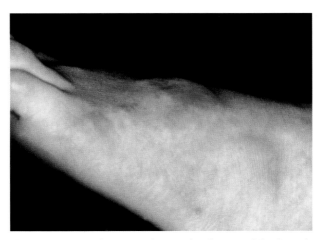

Figure 10.1 Granuloma annulare on the dorsum of the foot of a diabetic patient.

Skin lesions
Three specific skin lesions are seen in diabetes mellitus:
- diabetic dermopathy
- necrobiosis lipoidica diabeticorum
- diabetic bullae (bullosis diabeticorum).

Diabetic dermopathy takes the form of painless brown papules on the shins. It results from trauma to the skin causing microangiopathic changes in the capillaries (Figure 10.2). The lesions do not ulcerate, but undergo fibrosis leaving shallow scars. Evidence of other microangiopathic complications, such as retinopathy, nephropathy and neuropathy, is usually present.

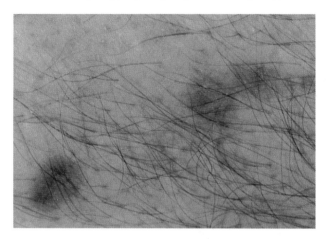

Figure 10.2
Diabetic dermopathy in a man with diabetes mellitus.

Necrobiosis lipoidica diabeticorum. The lesions of necrobiosis lipoidica diabeticorum start as scaly papules on the anterior aspect of one or both legs, but are occasionally found on the hands, forearms, abdomen and, rarely, the face. The lesions are painless and often progress to form large yellow sclerotic plaques with a purple periphery (Figure 10.3). Ulceration may occur. Over a period of years the plaques become fibrosed and atrophic. The characteristic histological appearance is one of degeneration (necrobiosis) of collagen in the presence of microangiopathy of the skin capillaries, with a central area of lipid-like material.

It is more often seen in women than in men and usually presents in adolescence. Although necrobiosis lipoidica diabeticorum is more commonly seen in patients with IDDM, up to 30% of cases may occur in non-diabetic individuals with impaired glucose tolerance or a family history of diabetes. The condition may, therefore, be a marker for the later development of overt diabetes mellitus.

There is no known effective treatment, although skin grafting has been used to try and improve the cosmetic appearance in severe cases.

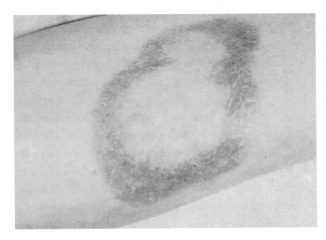

Figure 10.3
Necrobiosis lipoidica diabeticorum on the shin of a young woman with IDDM.

Diabetic bullae are intra-epidermal bullae that are most commonly seen in young, male IDDM patients with long-standing diabetes mellitus. The lesions are often seen in patients with chronic peripheral neuropathy. Diabetic bullae may be seen on the fingers and toes, and occasionally on the hands or feet.

Limited joint mobility (diabetic cheiroarthropathy)

Glycosylation of the palmar fascia and peri-articular tissue may cause stiffness in the hands. At an early stage, patients are unable to hyperextend the metacarpophalangeal joints. At a later stage, the condition can be demonstrated clinically by the failure of the two palms to touch each other when the hands are opposed – the so-called 'prayer' sign.

Patients with limited joint mobility usually have IDDM, and up to 30% of all IDDM patients have been reported to show this abnormality to some degree. In itself, it is of no real clinical importance, but its presence may indicate that other microangiopathic abnormalities may be present in the eye, kidney and peripheral nerves.

CHAPTER 11
Future trends

The prevalence of diabetes mellitus is increasing worldwide; in most non-white populations living in a Western culture, the prevalence of diabetes mellitus in the adult population is in the range of 15–20% (2–3 times that of the white population). When one considers that diabetes mellitus is the leading cause of blindness, kidney disease and amputations, and is associated with a 2–4-fold increased risk of cardiovascular disease, it is imperative that treatment strategies are developed and implemented to curb this devastating disease and its consequences.

Understanding the contributions of genetics and the environment

Individuals with IDDM and NIDDM have underlying genetic susceptibilities that predispose them to the development of their clinical disease. A major goal of the next decade will be to determine what these genetic factors are and how they interact with the environment.

The autoimmune form of diabetes, IDDM, is associated with certain HLA class II haptotypes which confer high risk for developing the disease. There are, however, other haptotypes (DQb1 0602) that confer protection against developing IDDM. These molecules are involved in presenting antigens to T cells. When an environmental factor interacts with the HLA class II haptotypes in a susceptible individual, an autoimmune response is triggered. That autoimmune response is marked by the generation of autoantibodies directed against insulin, glutamic acid decarboxylase (GAD), islet cell antibodies (ICA) 512 and many other molecules. The autoimmune response destroys the β-cells of the pancreas.

The genetic basis of NIDDM is far less clear. Although there is little insight into the mechanism responsible for the deficient β-cell reserve, it is known that factors, such as central obesity, physical inactivity and Western cultural influences, cause insulin resistance. Furthermore, the cascade responsible for intracellular insulin action can be inhibited by many metabolic factors. It should therefore be possible to determine how to decrease insulin resistance by modifying some of the events and factors involved.

Prevention of diabetes

Enough is known about the interaction of environmental and genetic factors in both IDDM and NIDDM that clinical trials are being undertaken to attempt to prevent them.

Individuals at high risk of developing IDDM can be identified by the presence of one or more autoantibodies and a decreased first phase insulin response to intravenous glucose. One prevention trial involves the administration of oral nicotinamide to these high-risk individuals to see if it delays or prevents the development of IDDM. Another, more complex trial involves the administration of small doses of parenteral insulin to see if the autoimmune process can be desensitized and stopped. It will, however, be several years before the results of these trials are available. In any event, it seems likely that IDDM will be amenable to preventive therapy within a decade.

The pathophysiology of NIDDM is very different from IDDM. Different strategies are being explored to prevent its development. The primary focus is to decrease insulin resistance. Thus, programmes that attempt to change lifestyle (e.g. diet, exercise), as well as those utilizing drugs such as acarbose, metformin or thiazolidenediones, are being proposed to treat individuals with impaired glucose tolerance to determine if the conversion to NIDDM can be prevented or delayed. More information about the β-cell abnormalities will probably be necessary before additional types of preventative trials can be initiated.

New treatments for hyperglycaemia

Many new agents are being investigated to determine their effectiveness in improving glycaemia in NIDDM. These agents can be classified into those which act through the gastrointestinal tract by increasing meal-mediated and basal insulin secretion, those which act by decreasing hepatic glucose production, and those which act by increasing the uptake and utilization of glucose by peripheral tissues.

Among the more promising agents are glucagon-like peptide 1 which is a gastrointestinal hormone, a variety of drugs that act on the ATP-dependent potassium channel of the β-cell to increase insulin secretion, and the thiazolidenediones which increase insulin action within insulin-sensitive cells by a variety of mechanisms.

Insulin analogues, such as Lys pro-insulin, are being developed. These analogues have a more rapid onset of action (within 15 minutes) and a shorter duration of action, and may reduce postprandial hypoglycaemia.

Agents to prevent end-organ damage. The results of the Diabetes Control and Complications Trial and many other smaller studies have shown that hyperglycaemia is responsible for the microvascular and neuropathic complications of diabetes mellitus. Several mechanisms have been proposed to explain the pathogenesis by which hyperglycaemia causes end-organ damage. These include:

- the aldose reductase pathway
- non-enzymatic glycosylation and advanced glycosylation end products
- alteration in tissue redox potential
- diacylglycerol protein kinase C pathway.

The aldose reductase pathway provides for a marked increase in sorbitol concentration within the cell when hyperglycaemia is present. Associated changes include a decrease in myoinositol and a reduction in sodium-potassium ATPase activity. This mechanism has been implicated in the development of cataracts, neuropathy and, possibly, retinopathy. A number of drugs to inhibit the aldose reductase pathway have been developed and used in clinical trials. At present, the clinical benefits in neuropathy have been minimal and in retinopathy non-existent. However, newer and more potent agents are being developed and tested.

Glycation of proteins and the production of advanced glycosylation end products (AGEs) occur during hyperglycaemia. In many studies in experimental diabetes, AGEs have been implicated as having pathogenic potential in the development of both microvascular and atherosclerotic disease. A simple chemical, aminoguanidine, prevents the formation of AGEs and has been shown in animal models to reduce vascular complications. Clinical trials of aminoguanidine are under way in patients with diabetes mellitus to determine whether microvascular and macrovascular disease can be reduced.

Key references

GENERAL

American Diabetes Association. Clinical Practice Recommendations 1996. *Diabetes Care* 1996;19(suppl 1):S1–118.

St Vincent Joint Task Force for Diabetes. *Department of Health and British Diabetes Association Report*. London: HMSO, 1995:1–31.

WHO Study Group. *Diabetes mellitus*. WHO Technical Report Series No 727. Geneva: WHO, 1985.

EPIDEMIOLOGY

Harris MJ, Hadden WC, Knowler WC, Bennett PH. Prevalence of diabetes and impaired glucose tolerance and plasma glucose levels in US population aged 20–74 years. *Diabetes* 1986;36:523–534.

Karoven M, Tuomilehto J, Libman I, La Porte R. A review of the recent epidemiological data on the worldwide incidence of Type 1 (insulin-dependent) diabetes mellitus. *Diabetologia* 1993;36:883–892.

WHAT IS IDDM ?

Ah-Chuan T, Eisenbarth GS. Natural history of IDDM. *Diabetes Rev* 1993;1:1–14.

Atkinson MA, MacLaren NK. The pathogenesis of insulin-dependent diabetes mellitus. *N Engl J Med* 1994; 331:1428–1436.

WHAT IS NIDDM ?

Haffner SM. The insulin resistance syndrome revisited. *Diabetes Care* 1996;19:275–277.

Lebovitz HE, Banerji MA, Chaiken RL. The relationship between type II diabetes and syndrome *X*. *Curr Opin Endocrinol Diabetes* 1995;2:307–312.

Yki-Jarvinen H. Pathogenesis of non-insulin dependent diabetes mellitus. *Lancet* 1994;343:91–95.

DIAGNOSIS OF IDDM AND NIDDM

Davies MJ, Gray IP. Impaired glucose tolerance. *BMJ* 1996;312:264–265.

WHO Expert Committee. *Second report on diabetes mellitus*. WHO Technical Report Series No 646. Geneva: WHO, 1980.

TREATMENT OF IDDM

Campbell IW. The optimal use of modern insulins. *Practitioner* 1994;238:46–52.

Ratner RE. Rational insulin management of insulin-dependent diabetes. In: Leslie RDG, Robbins DC, eds. *Diabetes: clinical science in practice*. Cambridge: Cambridge University Press, 1995:434–449.

TREATMENT OF NIDDM

Alberti KGMM, Gries FA et al. A desktop guide for the management of non-insulin dependent diabetes mellitus (NIDDM): an update. *Diabetic Med* 1994;11:899–909.

Bailey CJ, Turner RC. Metformin. *N Engl J Med* 1996;334:574–579.

Campbell IW. Efficacy and limitations of sulphonylureas and metformin. In: Bailey CJ, Flatt PR, eds. *New antidiabetic drugs*. Nischimura, Japan: Smith-Gordon, 1990:33–51.

Lebovitz HE. Stepwise and combination drug therapy for the treatment of NIDDM. *Diabetes Care* 1994; 17:1542–1544.

Shiasson J-L, Josse RG et al. The efficacy of acarbose in the treatment of patients with non-insulin-dependent diabetes mellitus. *Ann Int Med* 1994;121:928–935.

UK Prospective Diabetes Study 16. Overview of 6 years' therapy of type II diabetes: a progressive disease. *Diabetes* 1995;44:1249–1258.

Williams G. Management of non-insulin dependent diabetes mellitus. *Lancet* 1994;343:95–100.

COMPLICATIONS OF DIABETES MELLITUS AND THEIR MANAGEMENT

Campbell IW. Diabetic autonomic neuropathy. In: Tattersall RB, Gale EM, eds. *Diabetes: clinical management.* Edinburgh: Churchill Livingstone, 1990:307–320.

Dean JD, Durrington PN. Treatment of diabetic dyslipoproteinaemia in diabetes mellitus. *Diabetic Med* 1996;13:297–312.

Flanagan DW. Current management of established diabetic eye disease. *Eye* 1993;7:302–308.

Lein ME. Preventing amputation in the patient with diabetes. *Diabetes Care* 1995;18:1383–1393.

Mogensen CE, Keane WF et al. Prevention of diabetic renal disease with special reference to microalbuminuria. *Lancet* 1995;346:1080–1084.

Moser M, Ross H. The treatment of hypertension in diabetic patients. *Diabetes Care* 1993;16:542–547.

Stevens MJ, Feldman EL, Greene DA. The aetiology of diabetic neuropathy: the combined roles of metabolic and vascular defects. *Diabetic Med* 1995;12:566–579.

The Diabetes Control and Complications Trial Research Group. The effect of intensive treatment of diabetes on the development and progression of long-term complications in insulin-dependent diabetes mellitus. *N Engl J Med* 1993;329:977–986.

Wingard DL, Ferrara A, Barrett-Connor EL. Is insulin really a heart disease risk factor. *Diabetes Care* 1995; 18:1299–1304.

Young MJ, Breddy JL et al. The prediction of diabetic neuropathic foot ulceration using vibration perception thresholds. *Diabetes Care* 1994;6:557–560.

HYPOGLYCAEMIA AND DIABETIC KETOACIDOSIS

Cranston ICP, Amiel SA. Hypoglycaemia. In: Leslie RDG, Robbins DC, eds. *Diabetes: clinical science in practice.* Cambridge: Cambridge University Press, 1995:375–391.

Lebovitz HE. Diabetic ketoacidosis. *Lancet* 1995;345:767–772.

DIABETES AND THE SKIN

Boyd SG, Innes SM, Campbell IW. Skin manifestations of diabetes mellitus. *Practitioner* 1982;226:253–254.

Munro DW. Dermatological problems in diabetes. In: Besser GM, Bodansky HJ, Cudworth AG, eds. *Clinical diabetes.* London: Gower Medical Publishing, 1988:26.1–26.6

FUTURE TRENDS

Steel JM. What next in the treatment of diabetes? *Practitioner* 1996;240:116–119.